HERPES
PATIENT ADVOCATE

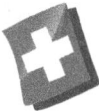

HealthScouter
WWW.HEALTHSCOUTER.COM

HealthScouter.com - Equity Press
5055 Canyon Crest Drive
Riverside, California 92507

www.healthscouter.com

Purchasing this book entitles you to free updates at www.healthscouter.com/Herpes

Edited By: Shana McKibbin

Includes Herpes Simplex Viruses from Wikipedia http://en.wikipedia.org/wiki/Herpes

HealthScouter Herpes: Genital Herpes Symptoms and Genital Herpes Treatment: Herpes Patient Advocate Guide

ISBN 978-1-60332-083-2

Important

NEVER DISREGARD PROFESSIONAL MEDICAL ADVICE, OR DELAY SEEKING IT, BECAUSE OF SOMETHING YOU HAVE READ IN THIS BOOK. ALWAYS SEEK PROFESSIONAL MEDICAL ADVICE BEFORE ACTING UPON INFORMATION READ IN THIS BOOK.

HealthScouter and Equity Press do not provide medical advice. The contents of this book are for informational purposes only and are not intended to substitute for professional medical advice, diagnosis or treatment. Always seek advice from a qualified physician or health care professional about any medical concern, and do not disregard professional medical advice because of anything you may read in this book or on a HealthScouter Web site. The views of individuals quoted in this book are not necessarily those of HealthScouter or Equity Press.

While this book is intended to be a medium for the exchange of information and ideas, it is not meant in any way to be a substitute for sound medical advice; neither should it be viewed as a trusted source of such advice. The views expressed in these messages are not those of any qualified medical association, and the publisher is not responsible for the validity of the information communicated herein or for consequences that may arise from acting upon this information. The publisher is not responsible for any content found in the book that may be deemed offensive, inappropriate, inaccurate or medically unsound. The information you find here is only for the purpose of discussion and should not be the basis for any medical decision. The content is not intended to be a substitute for professional medical advice, diagnosis or treatment.

The information presented is not to be considered complete, nor does it contain all medical resource information that may be relevant, and therefore it is not intended to be a substitute for seeking medical treatment and/or appropriate care.

By reading this book and parts of the Web site, you agree under all circumstances to hold harmless, and to refrain from seeking remedy from, the owners of this book. The publisher shall disclaim all liability to you for damages, costs or expenses, including legal and medical fees, related to your reliance on anything derived from this book or Web site or its contents. Furthermore, Equity Press assumes no liability for any and all claims arising out of the said use, regardless of the cause, effects, or fault.

Equity Press and HealthScouter do not endorse any company or product, and listing on the HealthScouter Web site is not linked to corporate sponsorship. We do not make a claim to being comprehensive or up to date. If you would like to recommend information to include in this book, please contact us – we would be very happy to hear from you.

Purchasing this book entitles you to free updates as they are available. Please register your book at www.healthscouter.com

TABLE OF CONTENTS

INTRODUCTION AND MOTIVATION

Dear Reader,

I like to think of myself as a polite, well-reasoned person. I rarely speak out or complain. When a waitress spills something on me, or if my meal is cold—or if I'm overcharged—I generally try to be as polite as possible. I don't like to make very many waves. I often secretly hope that the manager will hear about my predicament and come out and offer me a free meal, or something similar. I generally hope that my polite and respectful demeanor pays off. And it does happen from time to time. You know, I think many people are brought up to believe that this is just good manners. It's how you're supposed to behave. And if you knew me personally, I think you'd agree that I'm generally pretty reserved. Of course my wife may raise an objection or two (!), but I really believe that it's important to treat others as you would like to be treated. We're talking about the golden rule here—it works well and it applies to almost every life circumstance.

But I have to admit that when it comes to my health, or the health of someone I care about—all bets are off. I want to know what's going on—when, why, where, and how. And I make these feelings known. I tend to get downright assertive. It's just something I feel very strongly about. And I feel that when you are in a hospital, or if you're brushing up against the healthcare system, that you should feel the same way. It's unfamiliar turf, and the professionals who work in this system often take advantage of their positions. They may use some jargon to hide the whole truth— or they may say something without checking to make sure you understand completely. They may present the options that are best for them, perhaps the most profitable or convenient. Now I'm not saying this goes on everywhere. There are many professionals in the business of health who go out of their way to make sure you have the best care. And I'm not suggesting that you should become a bully, or purposefully annoying—absolutely not. But I am suggesting that I think it's OK for you to step outside of your typical comfort zone, and put on your patient advocate hat. Because you, the patient or patient advocate, care the most about your care—not the medical system or healthcare providers.

HealthScouter was created to help patients become better advocates for their own medical care. Because when it comes to your healthcare, the stakes are high. There are none higher. And healthcare is one area where consumers (us, the sick people) are notoriously unaware of their options. And that's why I'm publishing these books. To help you understand your options, and to help you get the best care possible. I want to help you become a better advocate for yourself and for your loved ones.

It's my sincere hope that you can take this book with you to the hospital, to be read in the waiting room or by the bedside—and when you see a relevant patient comment you can use this book to ask questions of your health care providers. My advice: Ask lots of questions! Providers are busy people who generally go about their business with little questioning, delivering care as they see fit—making quick decisions—and again, nobody is going to care as much about your health as you. So now, more than ever, you need tools at your disposal to get the best care possible. One of the tools at your disposal is this HealthScouter book and the material within. You need to be armed with questions, and you need to ask questions all of the time. And so the difficult part is now to understand the right questions to ask.

That brings me to an explanation of how these books are structured. HealthScouter books include a number of what we call patient comments. These patient comments are summaries of what people have experienced. They're first hand accounts of what you may expect. These experiences effectively help you "catch up," and understand what outcomes are possible. They expose you to the treatments are available, and provide insight as to potential outcomes. They help you understand what other people are doing. So if you find yourself stuck feeling like you're receiving substandard medical care—or if you need a push to broach the subject, you can take this book to your provider and say, "Hey, I read here that another patient had this treatment—is that an option for me? If not, Why?" I believe that other peoples' experience is the most valuable way for you to formulate and build a list of good questions for your healthcare providers.

That notion is at the core of the HealthScouter philosophy.

So HealthScouter, by providing patient comments about a particular medical condition, will help expose you to what other people have experienced about a particular medical problem. If you know what other people have experienced, you can better understand what your options are. You'll be better informed and you'll have some questions to ask—it'll be like you've had access to dozens of other people who have gone through the same thing you're going through. And so armed, maybe you'll be able to move through your condition and get back on the road to health, and maybe you'll be able to do this with more grace than I have. And that is my sincere wish.

It's also my wish that perhaps when a doctor or nurse sees this little blue book, that they'll think twice about the care they're about to provide—knowing that the owner is a little bit better prepared, a little bit better armed—and yes, maybe even downright assertive.

I hope this book helps.

Yours truly,

Jim Stewart

San Diego, California

HOW TO USE THIS BOOK

The purpose of HealthScouter is to help you understand your medical condition as quickly and easily as possible. We believe this can best be accomplished by reading about other people and their experiences negotiating their health and care. We try to leave out complicated medical jargon. And we've spent a considerable amount of time structuring this book so that it's easy to use. It's important to know that this is not the sort of book you read from beginning to end. Of course you may do so, but this book is more meaningful if you flip through quickly and scan for applicable material. Again, it's all about the patient commentary: The darkly shaded comments ▰ indicate one patient initiating a new discussion, and the light or clear comments ▱ are other comments associated with that same condition. So you should begin by looking for information from other patients who are experiencing the same aspect of the same medical condition that you studying. You can do this quickly by scanning through the book, focusing on the dark shaded comment boxes. By scanning the patient comments you'll find information about various aspects of a condition, all grouped together, in an easy-to-read format. In this way you can immediately begin reading about other patients and their experiences with your particular medical condition – and you can benefit immediately from their experiences.

INTRODUCTION TO HERPES

Herpes simplex virus 1 and 2 (HSV-1 and HSV-2) are two species of the herpes virus family, Herpesviridae, which cause infections in humans.[1] Eight members of herpes virus infect humans to cause a variety of illnesses including cold sores, chickenpox or varicella, shingles or herpes zoster (VZV), cytomegalovirus (CMV), and various cancers, and can cause brain inflammation (encephalitis). All viruses in the herpes family produce life-long infections.

They are also called Human Herpes Virus 1 and 2 (HHV-1 and HHV-2) and are neurotropic and neuroinvasive viruses; they enter and hide in the human nervous system, accounting for their durability in the human body. HSV-1 is commonly associated with herpes outbreaks of the face known as cold sores or fever blisters, whereas HSV-2 is more often associated with genital herpes.

An infection by a herpes simplex virus is marked by watery blisters in the skin or mucous membranes of the mouth, lips or genitals.[1] Lesions heal with a scab characteristic of herpetic disease. However, the infection is persistent and symptoms may recur periodically as outbreaks of sores near the site of original infection. After the initial, or primary, infection, HSV becomes latent in the cell bodies of nerves in the area. Some infected people experience sporadic episodes of viral reactivation, followed by transportation of the virus via the nerve's axon to the skin, where virus replication and shedding occurs.[2]

Herpes is contagious if the carrier is producing and shedding the virus. This is especially likely during an outbreak but possible at other times. There is no cure yet, but there are treatments which reduce the likelihood of viral shedding.

How can you pass the herpes virus to someone else when you're not having an outbreak?

By "asymptomatic shedding" during sex, kissing and/or oral sex. Basically means that the virus is active in one partner but they have no outward symptoms - bumps, sores etc. Skin to skin contact can pass it on. Condoms reduce the risk and suppressive medicine helps reduce the risk even more.

TRANSMISSION

HSV is transmitted during close contact with an infected person who is shedding virus from the skin, in saliva or in secretions from the genitals. This horizontal transmission of the virus is more likely to occur when sores are present, although viral shedding, and therefore transmission, does occur in the absence of visible sores.[3] In addition, vertical transmission of HSV may occur between mother and child during childbirth, which can be fatal to the infant.[4] The immature immune system of the child is unable to defend against the virus and even if treated, the infection can result in inflammation of the brain (encephalitis) that may cause brain damage. Transmission occurs when the infant passes through the birth canal, but the risk of infection is reduced if there are no symptoms or exposed blisters during delivery. The first outbreak after exposure to HSV is commonly more severe than future outbreaks, as the body has not had a chance to produce antibodies; this first outbreak carries a low (~1%) risk of developing aseptic meningitis.[1]

> *A guy I know had a cold sore on his lip and used a razor to shave around it. I used that razor on my vagina and two days later a sore showed up. Can I get herpes from that razor?*

Depends how soon after he used the razor that you did. The herpes simplex virus does not survive for long outside the body. If you used the razor immediately after him, there is a chance of transmission but it is unlikely.

How can someone get genital herpes when they are still a virgin?

Herpes can be spread simply by kissing someone on the mouth... also by touching a herpes sore and then touching someone else. It thrives best from direct skin to skin contact but can be spread by touching the sore and immediately touching someone else...just not as easily. So yes, you can get herpes still being a virgin.

Can someone get herpes from makeup, lipstick eye makeup?

I would say yes for herpes type 1, if the person has an active blister and you use it immediately after they applied the lipstick and touched the sore and then you used it. As for the mascara and other things, probably not. Mascara could infect if the person has a sty. Makeup I would say yes if the sore is on the face and then you use it. The virus is very contagious when active. You can spread it to your eyes too if you rub with your hands then rub your eyes.

Almost a month and a half ago I was diagnosed with herpes. I have HSV-1. I have met another guy who is interested in dating me and I did do the smart thing and tell him as soon as I could before the relationship got to serious. He is a real man about this he wants to get a better understanding of it and so do I. I have done a lot of research but what I'm looking for I haven't found. I know I cannot have sex which I do not plan to do for a years to come. What are limitations on sexual activity like if I kiss someone can I spread it. I know it can be spread through skin/ sexual fluid contact and when an outbreak occurs. I want to go about this smart in my future relationships and not put anyone else through like my ex did to me.

I caught HSV-1 about three years ago. At first I was devastated, I had it on my genitals and lips. I was having outbreaks about once a month at first. I started taking Valtrex 500mg once a day and this stuff works wonders for me. I have been in a relationship for a couple years now and my girlfriend hasn't caught it yet. There is always a risk that you could spread it put you have to let *your partner know. If he truly loves you he will understand. It's been over a year since I had an outbreak and when it occurs, it's real minor. When an outbreak occurs I increase to 1000MG a day for 3 days and it's gone in a week. It doesn't bother me that I have it now since it's under control.*

MICROBIOLOGY

Viral Structure

Animal herpes viruses all share some common properties. The structure of herpes viruses consists of a relatively large double-stranded, linear DNA genome encased within an icosahedral protein cage called the capsid, which is wrapped in a lipid bilayer called the envelope. The envelope is joined to the capsid by means of a tegument. This complete particle is known as the virion.[5] HSV-1 and HSV-2 each contain at least 74 genes (or open-reading frames, ORFs) within their genomes,[6] although speculation over gene crowding allows as many as 84 unique protein coding genes by 94 putative ORFs.[7] These genes encode a variety of proteins involved in forming the capsid, tegument and envelope of the virus, as well as controlling the replication and infectivity of the virus. These genes and their functions are summarized in the table below.

The genomes of HSV-1 and HSV-2 are complex, and contain two unique regions called the long unique region (U_L) and the short unique region (U_S). Of the 74 known ORFs, U_L contains 56 viral genes, whereas U_S contains only 12.[6] Transcription of HSV genes is catalyzed by RNA polymerase II of the infected host.[6] Immediate early genes, which encode proteins that regulate the expression of early and late viral genes, are the first to be expressed following infection. Early gene expression follows, to allow the synthesis of enzymes involved in DNA replication and the production of certain envelope glycoproteins. Expression of late genes occurs last; this group of genes predominantly encodes proteins that form the virion particle.[6]

Five proteins from (U_L) form the viral capsid; UL6, UL18, UL35, UL38 and the major capsid protein UL19.[5]

What are the causes of viral herpes? Is it because of the Chicken Pox Virus remaining latent in the body?

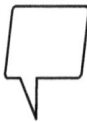

There are basically three forms of herpes virus: Simplex 1; Simplex 2 and Herpes Zoster. The scientific community may argue that there are variants within those types but that is a technicality.

Simplex 1 mainly affects the area around the mouth and Simplex 2 mainly affects the genitals but they can both affect either area.

Herpes Zoster is the chicken pox variety that remains dormant in the body and can emerge at times of stress in the form of shingles, usually on the front and back of the torso. It is also contagious and can cause chicken pox in people who have not previously had it.

Cellular Entry

Entry of HSV into the host cell involves interactions of several glycoproteins on the surface of the enveloped virus, with receptors on the surface of the host cell. The envelope covering the virus particle, when bound to specific receptors on the cell surface, will fuse with the host cell membrane and create an opening, or pore, through which the virus enters the host cell.

The sequential stages of HSV entry are analogous to those of other viruses. At first, complementary receptors on the virus and the cell surface bring the viral and cell membranes into proximity. In an intermediate state, the two membranes begin to merge, forming a hemifusion state. Finally, a stable entry pore is formed through which the viral envelope contents are introduced to the host cell.[12] In the case of a herpes virus, initial interactions occur when a viral envelope glycoprotein called glycoprotein C (gC) binds to a cell surface particle called heparan sulfate. A second glycoprotein, glycoprotein D (gD), binds specifically to a receptor called the herpes virus entry mediator receptor (HVEM) and provides a strong, fixed attachment to the host cell. These interactions bring the membrane surfaces into mutual proximity and allow for other glycoproteins embedded in the viral envelope to interact with other cell surface molecules. Once bound to the HVEM, gD changes its conformation and interacts with viral glycoproteins H (gH) and L (gL), which form a complex. The interaction of these membrane proteins results in the hemifusion state. Afterward, gB interaction with the gH/gL complex creates an entry pore for the viral capsid.[12] Glycoprotein B interacts with glycosaminoglycans on the surface of the host cell.

Genetic Inoculation

After the viral capsid enters the cellular cytoplasm, it is transported to the cell nucleus. Once attached to the nucleus at a nuclear entry pore, the capsid ejects its DNA contents via the capsid portal. The capsid portal is formed by twelve copies of portal protein, UL6, arranged as a ring; the proteins contain a leucine zipper sequence of amino acids which allow them to adhere to each other.[13] Each icosahedral capsid contains a single portal, located in one vertex.[14][15] The DNA exits the capsid in a single linear segment.[16]

Replication

Following infection of a cell, herpes virus proteins, called immediate-early, early, and late, are produced. Research using flow cytometrys on another member of the herpes virus family, KSHV, indicates the possibility of an additional lytic stage, delayed-late.[17] These stages of lytic infection, particularly late lytic, are distinct from the latency stage; in the case of HSV-1, no protein products are detected during latency whereas, they are detected during the lytic cycle.

The early proteins transcribed are used in the regulation of genetic replication of the virus. On entering the cell, an α-TIF protein joins the viral particle and aids in immediate-early transcription. The virion host shutoff protein (VHS or UL41) is very important to viral replication.[9] This enzyme shuts off protein synthesis in the host, degrades host mRNA, helps in viral replication, and regulates gene expression of viral proteins. The viral genome immediately travels to the nucleus but the VHS protein remains in the cytoplasm.[18][19]

The late proteins are used in to form the capsid and the receptors on the surface of the virus. Packaging of the viral particles— including the genome, core and the capsid - occurs in the nucleus of the cell. Here, concatemers of the viral genome are separated by cleavage and are placed into pre-formed capsids. HSV-1 undergoes a process of primary and secondary envelopment. The primary envelope is acquired by budding into the inner nuclear membrane of the cell. This then fuses with the outer nuclear membrane releasing a naked capsid into the cytoplasm. The virus acquires its final envelope by budding into cytoplasmic vesicles.[20]

Latent Infection

HSV may persist in a quiescent but persistent form known as latent infection, notably in neural ganglia.[1] During latent infection of a cell, HSV express Latency Associated Transcript (LAT) RNA. LAT is known to regulate the host cell genome and interferes with natural cell death mechanisms. By maintaining the host cells, LAT expression preserves a reservoir of the virus, which allows later recurrences to produce further infections.

A protein found in neurons may bind to herpes virus DNA and regulate latency. Herpes virus DNA contains a gene for a protein called ICP4, which is an important transactivator of genes associated with lytic infection in HSV-1.[21] Elements surrounding the gene for ICP4 bind a protein known as the human neuronal protein Neuronal Restrictive Silencing Factor (NRSF) or human Repressor Element Silencing Transcription Factor (REST). When bound to the viral DNA elements, histone deacytalization occurs atop the ICP4 gene sequence to prevent initiation of transcription from this gene, thereby preventing transcription of other viral genes involved in the lytic cycle.[22][23] Another HSV protein reverses the inhibition of ICP4 protein synthesis. ICP0 dissociates NRSF from the ICP4 gene and thus prevents silencing of the viral DNA.[24]

The virus can be reactivated by other illnesses such as cold and influenza, eczema, emotional and physical stress, exposure to bright sunlight, gastric upset, fatigue or injury, and by menstruation.

How ill can herpes make you if you are a diabetic and have asthma.

The reason I'm asking is that I've just found out I have herpes type one and my boyfriend has both of the above.

We are reading everything we can but cannot find anyone who has suffered with herpes and all the above.

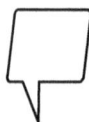

Well this is odd that I may be able to help you with this one after you replied to mine. I also have diabetes. My outbreak was pretty severe and although the doctor would not say so for sure, he felt that the diabetes may have played a role in how intense the outbreak was. Diabetes does make it harder to heal and sometimes make you more susceptible to other illnesses. He put my on a daily medication that will not interfere with the diabetic medication I take. It will reduce the amount of outbreaks I have and hopefully make the next outbreak less severe. Although they say they get lesser with each outbreak.

TREATMENT

"Current medically accepted methods of treating infections caused by the herpes virus are chemotherapeutic agents which are applied topically, injected or taken orally. Such treatment can often deal with the immediate infection but does not prevent a recurrence of the infection at a later date after the treatment has ceased."[25] Some attempts have been made to treat individuals affected with the herpes virus by treatment with light of the wavelength 660nm, as described in US Patent 5500009.[26] However, the present inventor was unable to achieve a significant clinical outcome or benefit at that wavelength.[25] Furthermore, according to US Patent # 2005234383, it has been established that "low intensity electromagnetic radiation of small bandwidth is effective in the treatment of infectious diseases, inflammatory-type diseases and other conditions, including the alleviation of pain."[25]

ALZHEIMER'S DISEASE

Scientists discovered a link between HSV-1 and Alzheimer's disease in 1979.[27] In the presence of a certain gene variation (APOE-epsilon4 allele carriers), HSV-1 appears to be particularly damaging to the nervous system and increases one's risk of developing Alzheimer's disease. The virus interacts with the components and receptors of lipoproteins, which may lead to the development of Alzheimer's disease.[28] This research identifies HSVs as the pathogen most clearly linked to the establishment of Alzheimer's.[29] Without the presence of the gene allele, HSV type 1 does not appear to cause any neurological damage and thus increase the risk of Alzheimer's.[30]

A 2008 study published in The Journal of Pathology,[31] has shown a striking localization of herpes simplex virus type 1 DNA within the beta-amyloid plaques that characterize Alzheimer's disease, and suggests that this virus is a major cause of the plaques and hence probably a significant aetiological factor in Alzheimer's disease.

HERPES SIMPLEX VIRUS 1 & 2

Herpes simplex (from the Greek ἕρπης /ˈerpis/) is a viral disease caused by herpes simplex viruses; both herpes simplex virus 1 (HSV-1) and herpes simplex virus 2 (HSV-2) cause herpes simplex. Infection with the herpes virus is categorized into one of several distinct disorders based on the site of infection. Oral herpes, the visible symptoms of which are colloquially called cold sores, infects the face and mouth. Oral herpes is the most common form of infection. Infection of the genitals, commonly known as herpes, is the second most common form of herpes. Other disorders such as herpetic whitlow, herpes gladiatorum, ocular herpes (keratitis), cerebral herpes infection encephalitis, Mollaret's meningitis, neonatal herpes, and possibly Bell's palsy are all caused by herpes simplex viruses.

Herpes viruses cycle between periods of active disease—presenting as blisters containing infectious virus particles—that last 2–21 days, followed by a remission period, during which the sores disappear. Genital herpes, however, is often asymptomatic, though viral shedding may still occur. After initial infection, the viruses move to sensory nerves, where they reside as life-long, latent viruses. Causes of recurrence are uncertain, though some potential triggers have been identified. Over time episodes of active disease reduce in frequency.

Herpes simplex is most easily transmitted by direct contact with a lesion or the body fluid of an infected individual. Transmission may also occur through skin-to-skin contact during periods of asymptomatic shedding. Barrier protection methods are the most reliable method of preventing transmission of herpes, but they merely reduce rather than eliminate risk. Oral herpes is easily diagnosed if the patient presents with visible sores or ulcers. Early stages of orofacial herpes and genital herpes are harder to diagnose; laboratory testing is usually required. Prevalence of HSV infections varies throughout the world. Poor hygiene, overcrowding, lower socioeconomic status, and birth in an undeveloped country have been identified as risk factors associated with increased HSV-1 childhood infection. Additional studies have identified other risk factors for both types of HSV.

There is currently no cure for herpes; no vaccine is currently available to prevent or eliminate herpes, although vaccines of varying effectiveness are currently in phase III trials. Also, treatments are available to reduce viral reproduction and shedding, prevent the virus from entering the skin, and alleviate the severity of symptomatic episodes.

Herpes simplex should not be confused with herpes zoster, which is a viral disease caused by varicella zoster virus.

Is Herpes Zoster infectious?

More contagious than infectious! It can cause chicken pox in someone who has not had it or it can trigger an attack of shingles in someone who has already had chicken pox. For that reason, it is best to keep the sores loosely covered to allow them to dry, but prevent contact.

I have herpes zoster and this is the first time for me to have it and I started to take medication (Valtrex) and I was looking on the internet for the causes of this and it said it can be from HIV and I have just got 2 weeks back my results for an HIV test which came out negative .I made that test after 5 month of the last time I had sex and it was unsecured. Could there be a probability that the result of HIV test was not correct?

What could be the reason for this please help do I have to make a new HIV test to make sure that it is negative.

Don't panic herpes zoster (shingles) only happens to people who have had chicken pox. It is normally an indication of a low state of general health and typically occurs at times of stress. That's why it often affects people with HIV, because their immune system is unable to fight back. However, there is absolutely no reason to think that having shingles is an indication of HIV - it happens to many people, sometimes without any evident reason.

Unpleasant though it is, this opportunistic virus just attacks people when they are down and the chances are that you will never have it again.

My mom had Shingles when she was in her 80's.... she is 94 now. It has nothing to do with HIV.

If I have unprotected sex with my girlfriend when she has a cold sore on her lip can I catch herpes even if we do not kiss?

Does anyone else here have back issues and find that their outbreaks seem to follow when the nerves are irritated??? I had a deep tissue massage yesterday, no sore, then woke up today with the start of it-full blown tonight, and, my last outbreak followed along my sciatic nerve and appeared after a day of bad sciatic pain in my sacrum.

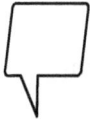

All this is true, the virus lives inside your nerves. That is why there is no cure for it, and you can't heal from it. So whenever your tissue weakens, the virus can travel up the nerves and then take over. Just like an infection can happen in a cut! Just keep your hands from your face, because it can go to your optic nerve and cause blindness. That is everything the doctor told me to do.

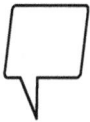

I always get them when I am stressed out or eating bad foods and not drinking enough water. Stay away from alcohol, etc. etc. Ask your doctor about Valtrex, because I think that is for people who break out like all the time.

I found two small bumps connected to each other...on my pubic bone region. The next day, they started to hurt and I noticed white tips...they look like pimples. I popped it but it hasn't gone down. I popped it again today and a little pus came out but mostly blood. It doesn't really hurt just aches a little bit like a pimple. Could this be a sign of herpes? Herpes is opened sores right? I'm hoping I'm just overanalyzing the situation. I've been with the same person for a year; the bumps

feels scarred when I put my finger over it but
there is no open sore...just two tiny holes where I
popped it. Do I have something to worry about?

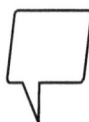

Sounds like ingrown hairs or to little pimples to me.

A little over three months ago I was in a
relationship and had unprotected sex. Within two
or three days I had an itching sensation in my
lower region. I immediately broke up with him
and refused to talk to him because I assumed he
had given me an STD, which he swears he has no
symptoms. I first thought it was a yeast infection
because I do get those often; however, the
medication didn't work. I later found little, I mean
TINY, whitish bumps around my labia which have
not gone away, popped, nor changed in size.
They are also not painful to the touch. I went to
the clinic to be examined for all STDs and they
said I was all clear. As I was still experiencing
pain, I went to my regular doctor who said I
had a UTI and gave me meds. A few days after
I finished the antibiotics, the pain and itching
returned. I guess my questions are: Has anyone
who has genital herpes experience non-stop
itching for over 3 or 4 months straight. Also, is it
possible to have herpes sores that never change

and simply stay there all the time? I don't fit what all the Web sites say about genital herpes; however, those are the typical textbook cases! Correct?

This does not sound like herpes. I think the clinic or your doctor would have identified any other type of infection so another question to ask yourself is - could this be an allergic reaction to new underwear, detergent, deodorant, soap or something else that you've recently started using/ wearing?

I pretty sure it isn't an allergic reaction to anything. I have just been thinking that my symptoms may be herpes because I have no clue as to what else it could be. Although my symptoms aren't like any typical herpes case, they did show up right after sex. Also, can antibiotics temporarily treat any pain caused by genital herpes? Thanks for the advice.

Antibiotics would only relieve pain by killing any bacteria that were causing the pain (unusual).

The only way to resolve this would be by proper medical analysis.

Did the doctor take swabs or do a blood test?
You say you were 'examined' but was that just a
visual examination? Did they culture for yeast or
bacteria?

Sometimes you have to speak up for your medical
rights and ask/demand. Especially if this is still
ongoing with you.

They did do a culture for bacteria at the STD
clinic. I told them to test for everything, but I
found out later everything apparently didn't
include the herpes virus (which is insane). The
doctor said they could only test for it if I was
having an outbreak. Three doctors have looked
at me but none have seen the little white bumps
that I see. They never go away nor change.
And I am always itching. Is this possible with
the herpes virus? I have even started taking
supplements such as L-lysine and vitamin C to
help with the virus but have not yet responded.
I am confused. When I get an opportunity I am
going to demand a blood test. Any thoughts on
the constant, painless to the touch, bumps and
constant itching? I mean not a day has gone by
in three months that I have not had either.

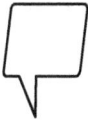

Sounds like it could be HPV and small warts. Don't panic. Just test for it and see. They look like you described.

Does HPV cause herpes?

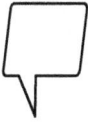

No, HPV and HSV (herpes) are two totally different viruses.

Some strains of HPV can cause genital warts, and others cause cervical dysplasia, which in the worst case scenario could develop into cervical cancer.

Please share with me the difference in the virus and why if both are sexually transmitted why does one show on the mouth and the other on the vagina?

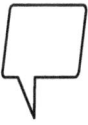

In short HSV-1 and 2 are very similar but 1 tends to favor the facial area whereas 2 tends to favor the genital area. However, they can swap places. The key is the initial site of infection. Someone who has an outbreak as a cold sore can re-infect themselves in the genital area and vice versa. With proper hygiene, an infection that starts in either area will always remain in that area. On its own, it does not migrate around the body - it has to be transferred by external means.

TRANSMISSION AND PREVENTION

Herpes is contracted through direct contact with an active lesion or body fluid of an infected person.[29] Herpes transmission occurs between discordant partners; a person with a history of infection (HSV seropositive) can pass the virus to an HSV seronegative person. The only way to contract herpes simplex virus 2 is through direct skin-to-skin contact with an infected individual. To infect a new individual, HSV travels through tiny breaks in the skin or mucous membranes in the mouth or genital areas. Even microscopic abrasions on mucous membranes are sufficient to allow viral entry.

HSV asymptomatic shedding occurs at some time in most individuals infected with herpes. It can occur more than a week before or after a symptomatic recurrence in 50% of cases.[30] Infected people that show no visible symptoms may still shed and transmit virus through their skin; asymptomatic shedding may represent the most common form of HSV-2 transmission.[30] Asymptomatic shedding is more frequent within the first 12 months of acquiring HSV. Concurrent infection with HIV increases the frequency and duration of asymptomatic shedding.[31] There are indications that some individuals may have much lower patterns of shedding, but evidence supporting this is not fully verified; no significant differences are seen in the frequency of asymptomatic shedding when comparing persons with 1 to 12 annual recurrences to those that have no recurrences.[30]

Antibodies that develop following an initial infection with a type of HSV prevent reinfection with the same virus type—a person with a history of orofacial infection caused by HSV-1 cannot contract herpes whitlow or a genital infection caused by HSV-1. In a monogamous couple, a seronegative female runs a greater than 30% per year risk of contracting an HSV infection from a seropositive male partner.[32] If an oral HSV-1 infection is contracted first, seroconversion will have occurred after 6 weeks to provide protective antibodies against a future genital HSV-1 infection.

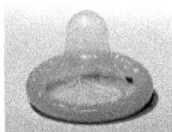

Barrier protection, such as a condom, can reduce the risk of herpes transmission.

For genital herpes, condoms are highly effective in limiting transmission of herpes simplex infection.[33][34] The virus cannot pass through latex, but a condom's effectiveness is somewhat limited on a public health scale by their limited use in the community,[35] and on an individual scale because the condom may not completely cover blisters on the penis of an infected male, or the base of the penis or testicles not covered by the condom may come into contact with free virus in vaginal fluid of an infected female. In such cases, abstinence from sexual activity or washing of the genitals after sex is recommended. The use of condoms or dental dams also limits the transmission of herpes from the genitals of one partner to the mouth of the other (or vice versa) during oral sex. When one partner has a herpes simplex infection and the other does not, the use of antiviral medication, such as valacyclovir, in conjunction with a condom, further decreases the chances of transmission to the uninfected partner.[3] Topical microbicides which contain chemicals that directly inactivate the virus and block viral entry are currently being investigated.[3] Vaccines for HSV are currently undergoing trials. Once developed, they may be used to help with prevention or minimize initial infections as well as treatment for existing infections.[36]

As with almost all sexually transmitted infections, women are more susceptible to acquiring genital HSV-2 than men.[37] On an annual basis, without the use of antivirals or condoms, the transmission risk of HSV-2 from infected male to female is approximately 8–10%.[32][38] This is believed to be due to the increased exposure of mucosal tissue to potential infection sites. Transmission risk from infected female to male is approximately 4–5% annually.[38] Suppressive antiviral therapy reduces these risks by 50%.[39] Antivirals also help prevent the development of symptomatic HSV in infection scenarios—meaning the infected partner will be seropositive but symptom free—by about 50%. Condom use also reduces the transmission risk by 50%.[33][34][40] Condom use is much more effective at preventing male to female transmission than vice-versa.[33] The effects of combining antiviral and condom use is roughly additive, thus resulting in approximately a 75% combined reduction in annual transmission risk. These figures reflect experiences with subjects having frequently-recurring genital herpes (>6 recurrences per year). Subjects with low recurrence rates and those with no clinical manifestations were excluded from these studies.

The risk of transmission from mother to baby is highest if the mother becomes infected at around the time of delivery (transmission risk 30 to 60%),[41][42] but the risk falls to 3% if it is a recurrent infection, and is less than 1% if there are no visible lesions.[43] To prevent neonatal infections, seronegative women are recommended to avoid unprotected oral-genital contact with an HSV-1 seropositive partner and conventional sex with a partner having a genital infection during the last trimester of pregnancy. A seronegative mother that contracts HSV at this time has up to a 57% chance of conveying the infection to her baby during childbirth, since insufficient time will have occurred for the generation and transfer of protective maternal antibodies before the birth of the child, whereas a woman seropositive for both HSV-1 and HSV-2 has around a 1–3% chance of transmitting infection to her infant.[44][45] Women that are seropositive for only one type of HSV are only half as likely to transmit HSV as infected seronegative mothers. Mothers infected with HSV are advised to avoid procedures that would cause trauma to the infant during birth (e.g., fetal scalp electrodes, forceps, and vacuum extractors) and, should lesions be present, to elect caesarean section to reduce exposure of the child to infected secretions in the birth canal.[3] The use of antiviral treatments, such as acyclovir, given from the 36th week of pregnancy limits HSV recurrence and shedding during childbirth, thereby reducing the need for caesarean section.[3]

HSV-2 infected individuals are at higher risk for acquiring HIV when practicing unprotected sex with HIV positive persons,[46] particularly during an outbreak with active lesions.[47]

If you have herpes and are pregnant, can the virus affect the baby when you have an amniocentesis?

No, the baby can only be affected when it passes through the birth canal. My herpes was not active when I delivered, but my OB-GYN will ONLY deliver babies by c-section if the mother is a carrier.

That is definitely a question to ask your doctor.

If my husband and I want to have a baby and I have herpes but he doesn't, what should I do?

My ex-wife and I both have genital herpes.

We have two beautiful children through natural childbirth. She was on Valtrex during her pregnancy and never had an outbreak.

The doctors assured us that the chances of passing it on were very slim and that they would stay on top of the situation.

The biggest risk is when the female does not have herpes, but contracts it in the third trimester of the process.

Talk with your doctors and voice your concerns, but by all means, if you want children, have them!

If I had a condom and it broke while having sex with a girl with herpes, would I necessarily get it?

Not necessarily. If she was not having an outbreak, the chances are slim.

If she was having an outbreak, she probably wouldn't be having sex with you, as it can be uncomfortable to say the least.

Even though you can pass the herpes virus on when not having an outbreak, it doesn't happen a lot. You will also find out that a condom isn't absolute protection for things like herpes, as it can be on other areas of the body. It could be on her thigh and you come in contact with her thigh against yours.

You'll know in a day or so if you caught it, more than likely, however some people carry the virus without ever having an outbreak.

To prevent outbreaks:

2,000mg of lysine daily works well, at least for me. Let your body rest from this high dosage occasionally. Other benefits of lysine: it has a mild function as a serotonin reuptake inhibitor, so may function as a mood enhancer as a side benefit.

Be careful about eating foods with high arginine content, and you should probably avoid libido enhancing formulas containing arginine. Turkey is the worst for me. Arginine is a libido stimulant, unfortunately, but if you do eat a high arginine food, take some lysine with it.

Avoid getting the area where you break out overly hot. A tanning bed can start an outbreak for me.

To stop outbreak in its tracks:

At first tingle or itch, IMMEDIATELY take your acyclovir or Valtrex and continue every couple of hours, along with four 1,000 tablet of lysine. If your symptoms subside, continue second day dropping down to prescribed acyclovir or Valtrex dosage, which is probably four times a day, accompanied each time by 4,000mg of lysine.

Do this even if symptoms have disappeared. This should stop the outbreak in its tracks. To be safe, you should probably continue drug dosage third day, and you can drop the lysine to 2,000mg.

For itching:

Cheap nail polish remover with acetone applied with a cotton pad or ball will stop itching though expect it to sting like heck for a couple of minutes. The relief will last for hours and for me is well worth the temporary discomfort. This was "prescribed" for me by a doctor back in the '60's, long before acyclovir had been invented.

For pain:

I use Aleve, but I would imagine Advil would work as well.

Feeling crummy:

You have an active virus. Treat yourself the same way you would if you had the flu. Get plenty of rest. Avoid alcohol!

My history:

I have had herpes for over 35 years, and do not recall it ever being in the genital area. It shows up as an area of itching, scaly blisters on my back about three inches below my waist.

During these 35 years I have never used protection, and have never passed it on. At this time I do not have sex when it is active. However, my husband of 20 years never contracted it from me, even though he insisted on having sex when I had an outbreak. I would insist, however, on covering the area with a large Band-Aid. THIS IS CERTAINLY NOT A RECOMMENDATION, just meant to reassure others that this disease can be no more than an occasional inconvenience for some people.

DIAGNOSIS

Primary orofacial herpes is readily identified by clinical examination of persons with no previous history of lesions and contact with an individual with known HSV-1 infection. The appearance and distribution of sores in these individuals typically presents as multiple, round, superficial oral ulcers, accompanied by acute gingivitis.[48] Adults with non-typical presentation are more difficult to diagnose. Prodromal symptoms that occur before the appearance of herpetic lesions help differentiate HSV symptoms from the similar symptoms of other disorders, such as allergic stomatitis. When lesions do not appear inside the mouth primary orofacial herpes is sometimes mistaken for impetigo, a bacterial infection. Common mouth ulcers (aphthous ulcer) also resemble intraoral herpes, but do not present a vesicular stage.[48]

Genital herpes can be more difficult to diagnose than oral herpes since most HSV-2-infected persons have no classical symptoms.[48] Further confusing diagnosis, several other conditions resemble genital herpes, including lichen planus, atopic dermatitis, and urethritis.[48] Laboratory testing is often used to confirm a diagnosis of genital herpes. Laboratory tests include: culture of the virus, direct fluorescent antibody (DFA) studies to detect virus, skin biopsy, and polymerase chain reaction (PCR) to test for presence of viral DNA. Although these procedures produce highly sensitive and specific diagnoses, their high costs and time constraints discourage their regular use in clinical practice.[48]

Serological tests for antibodies to HSV are rarely useful to diagnosis and not routinely used in clinical practice[48], but are important in epidemiological studies. Serologic assays cannot differentiate between antibodies generated in response to a genital versus an oral HSV infection, and as such cannot confirm the site of infection. Absence of antibody to HSV-2 does not exclude genital infection because of the increasing incidence of genital infections caused by HSV-1.

I have genital herpes. I have never noticed any signs of this before. I have had the same boyfriend for 9 months now and have not been with any other person in that time. Does this mean that he has cheated for sure? He says that he did not. My friend said some people have it for years before having signs. I don't know if he did this or not.

Also is there any kind of blood test you can get that tells you if you have it for sure? Because my boyfriend said he had one recently and it came back that he has it.

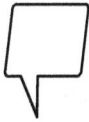

How were you diagnosed? By a visual exam, a swab culture? There is a blood test that detects antibodies to the virus. You should ask your doctor for a "type specific IgG" blood test. Herpeselect is a common name for one type done. DO NOT get an IgM test as that is not reliable.

If your partner has been tested ask to SEE the results. Has he ever had a cold sore which is herpes type 1. That could be transmitted to you via oral sex.

If you have a swab culture that is positive and a blood test that comes up negative that usually indicates that this is a new infection. If the blood test comes up positive also that indicates that you have had the virus about 3–4 months. (It takes that long generally for your body to produce antibodies that are detected in the blood test.)

Many people have it and don't know they have it. It does not automatically mean that your partner cheated on you.

Is there a possibility or what is the possibility of being infected with herpes from a routine haircut from a public barbershop?

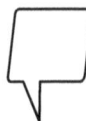

No.

What is the first sign of a person having herpes?

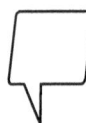

A burning/itching sensation followed within 24 hours by the eruption of a sore at the same location - around the mouth or the genitals. Seek medical attention immediately and avoid physical contact to avoid passing on the infection.

It often starts with a stinging or tingling sensation in your mouth area or genitals, and can be accompanied with flu like symptoms, fatigue or achiness. Herpes usually shows up anywhere from 2–21 days after initial exposure or sometimes can stay in hibernation for years. It is contracted from skin-to-skin contact, typically. Also, a herpes test is NOT included (here in the US) in the standard STD testing, you need to ask for it, how CRAZY is that...

DISORDERS

HSV infection causes several distinct medical disorders. Common infection of the skin or mucosa may affect the face and mouth (orofacial herpes), genitalia (genital herpes), or hands (herpes whitlow). More serious disorders occur when the virus infects and damages the eye (herpes keratitis), or invades the central nervous system, damaging the brain (herpes encephalitis). Patients with immature or suppressed immune systems, such as newborns, transplant recipients, or AIDS patients are prone to severe complications from HSV infections. HSV infection has also been associated with cognitive deficits of bipolar disorder,[1] and Alzheimer's disease,[2] although this is often dependent on the genetics of the infected person.

In all cases HSV is never removed from the body by the immune system. Following a primary infection, the virus enters the nerves at the site of primary infection, migrates to the cell body of the neuron, and becomes latent in the ganglion.[3] As a result of primary infection, the body produces antibodies to the particular type of HSV involved, preventing a subsequent infection of that type at a different site. In HSV-1 infected individuals, seroconversion after an oral infection will prevent additional HSV-1 infections such as whitlow, genital herpes, and keratitis. Prior HSV-1 seroconversion seems to reduce the symptoms of a later HSV-2 infection, although HSV-2 can still be contracted. Most indications are that an HSV-2 infection contracted prior to HSV-1 seroconversion will also immunize that person against HSV-1 infection.[4]

A few months back I was told I had herpes and that was it. My doctor didn't tell me much about it she just said that it was herpes.

The thing is it's on my pinky finger. I have never had an outbreak in any other area (mouth, vagina, anus, etc.), but a close friend of mine has informed me that I might have "herpetic whitlow"; she said that there are two types of herpes. Herpes simplex virus 1 and 2. HSV1 is when your body is only affected above the waistline, it is transmitted when touching an object especially when you lesion or wound is open. Herpes infection of the finger. It has nothing to do with sexual contact!!! the finger is the most common place to get infected cause you get it from touching anything that had the virus living on it...is this true? It sounds like exactly what's going on with me!!

My doctor also told me that I can get it from touching things which was "rare", that's why I assumed I had "regular" herpes.

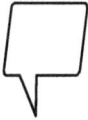

I was diagnosed seven years ago with genital herpes. I did a ton of research then. I have had only a few outbreaks all within the first couple years. All but one was in the genital area. I had one patch of blisters that broke out on the back of my calf. They eventually broke open and healed but it took a long time. The virus can occur anywhere in your body. It used to be true that HSV 1 was "above the waist" and type 2 was below but it is possible to spread either one to the opposite area. If you have a cold sore on your mouth and perform oral sex...you can acquire type 1 herpes, where type 2 is more common and vice versa. Just be very careful not to touch your face or eyes especially with the pinky that is affected and be sure to wash your hands often. That is probably a difficult place to keep it covered. I hope that helped a little.

RECURRENCE

Following active infection herpes viruses establish a latent infection in sensory and autonomic ganglia of the nervous system. The double-stranded DNA of the virus is incorporated into the cell physiology by infection of the nucleus of a nerve's cell body. HSV latency is static—no virus is produced—and is controlled by a number of viral genes, including Latency Associated Transcript (LAT).[18]

Many HSV infected people experience recurrence within the first year of infection.[3] Prodrome precedes development of lesions. Prodromal symptoms include tingling (paresthesia), itching, and pain where lumbosacral nerves innervate the skin. Prodrome may occur as long as several days or as short as a few hours before lesions develop. Beginning antiviral treatment when prodrome is experienced can reduce the appearance and duration of lesions in some individuals. During recurrence fewer lesions are likely to develop, lesions are less painful, and lesions heal faster (within 5–10 days without antiviral treatment), than those occurring during the primary infection.[3] Subsequent outbreaks tend to be periodic or episodic, occurring on average four to five times a year when not using antiviral therapy.

The causes of reactivation are uncertain, but several potential triggers have been documented. Physical or psychological stress can trigger an outbreak of herpes.[19] A recent study (2009) showed that a protein VP16 plays a key role in reactivation of the dormant virus.[20] Changes in the immune system during menstruation may play a role in HSV-1 reactivation.[21][22] Concurrent infections, such as viral upper respiratory tract infection or other febrile diseases, can cause outbreaks. Reactivation due to infection is the likely source of the historic terms cold sore and fever blister.

Other identified triggers include: local injury to the face, lips, eyes, or mouth, trauma, surgery, radiotherapy, and exposure to wind, ultraviolet light, or sunlight.[23][24][25][26][27]

The frequency and severity of recurrent outbreaks may vary greatly between patients. An immunity to the virus is built over time; immunocompromised individuals may experience episodes that are longer, more frequent and more severe. Antiviral medication has been proven to shorten the frequency and duration of outbreaks.[28] Outbreaks may occur at the original site of the infection or in close proximity to nerve endings that reach out from the infected ganglia. In the case of a genital infection, sores can appear at the original site of infection or near the base of the spine, the buttocks, back of the thighs.

I just want to know if herpes always clusters or can it show up as small scattered protruding bumps that itch but don't really hurt? I only could have been exposed to herpes like a month ago and I have these bumps on my thighs buttocks and around my armpits but none are clustered together and from what I can tell they don't look like herpes sores and they are very small about 5mm in diameter. Would my urine definitely burn if I had herpes or is that only a maybe, are there any definite symptoms to keep an eye out for?

I was diagnosed with herpes in April and I have had frequent ob's! My Dr put me on daily therapy but I still have had an outbreak. My question is could my frequent outbreaks be due to not having a spleen?? Which is the main organ of your immune system?

Anytime your immune system is compromised or weak, you are susceptible to outbreaks. Ask your doctor for ways to boost your immune system, daily vitamins would probably help.

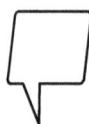

I contracted Type 1 genital herpes from my boyfriend giving me oral sex. I've always has a strong immune system (might get sick 1x a year at the most) but with all the stress from my job, I've always taken a prenatal vitamin (lots of B vitamins, plus if I'm going to get pregnant, it will be within the next two years), flaxseed oil gels, fiber chews and now I've started drinking this yogurt shot with L. Casei immunitants in the morning. It's really good and I don't handle dairy products very well, but I have no problems with this stuff! You can find it at any grocery store. I've even found it in a "light" formula. And just to be on the safe side, I continue taking my daily dose of Valtrex but will be switching to Acyclovir when that runs out. Acyclovir is cheaper ($4) and to me worth taking a pill everyday to control any outbreak that might occur. Although I've had only "1" outbreak, I still want to take a pill everyday to make sure. To me, it's not a hassle at all. We all take allergy medications to block out pollens and stuff so why not take a pill everyday to help control the outbreak. Some people on here might differ. I read on here that some only take meds when they have an outbreak. Hope you feel better!

It can take a few months to get your body regulated with the suppressive therapy. You will start to have less symptoms and then less worry. Lack of sleep several days in a row is my BIGGEST trigger...even being on suppressive for years. I will occasionally have one but it doesn't last as long.

TREATMENT

There is currently no cure that can eradicate herpes virus from the body, but antiviral medications can reduce the frequency, duration, and severity of outbreaks. Antiviral drugs also reduce asymptomatic shedding; it is believed asymptomatic HSV-2 viral shedding occurs on 10.8% of days per year in patients not undergoing antiviral treatment, versus 2.9% of days while on antiviral therapy.[30] Non-prescription analgesics can reduce pain and fever during initial outbreaks. Topical anesthetic treatments such as prilocaine, lidocaine or tetracaine can also relieve itching and pain.[81][82]

How can I get herpes cured? What type of medication do I apply to eliminate this epidemic?

You can be treated with Valtrex, which is probably the most popular, effective medication for Herpes. There are also other drugs, like acyclovir, which are less expensive and can be effective.

If you want to try other, non-prescription things, you can take Lysine, red marine algae as well as some topical things like DMSO cream and H-Balm. I have had luck with some of these things.

During the time I had my first few Herpes outbreaks, I had other new health issues pop up as well. I haven't seen anyone mention these issues but I can't help but wonder if anyone else had episodes of Vertigo or new acne when they first started having outbreaks... It's been 8 months since my first OB and 4 since I started daily suppressive meds. I haven't had Vertigo or acne for the past four months. Maybe it's just a coincidence but thought I would ask.

It is quite possible that the medication is causing both the vertigo and the acne. You should report these symptoms to your doctor.

Presumably you are taking a form of acyclovir which can produce these side-effects in some people.

I had the acne and vertigo while I was having outbreaks in the beginning. I don't have them anymore... I'm afraid that if I stop taking my suppressive meds those other issues come back as well.

These conditions are not normally associated with herpes but they are perhaps symptomatic of the low general state of health that allowed the herpes virus to attack your system.

So long as your general state of health is good, it is unlikely that you would get them again just because you back-off the medication.

I had extremely frequent acne when I first started having my outbreaks. For about two months, I had at least one new pimple every day. It started to calm down a bit after that. I never had anything like that before...even when I was a teenager! Maybe it's the stress on the body from the virus? I'm not sure if it's the meds that I'm taking for Herpes that has calmed the acne now that I'm outbreak free. I started daily meds after four months of outbreaks because I didn't know I had. At this point, I'm acne free. I hope you and your husband get there too!

I get regular outbreaks of the herpes on my buttocks left side why? And how can I make them less frequent it really gets me down, could there be another underlying reason why?

Is the spot you are getting them the initial spot of exposure? Meaning is this where the first outbreak occurred? If not the answer that I found was that because it lives in the sacral nerve it can come out anywhere along that nerve path. I get them on my but cheek as well but was not initially exposed there. There really isn't anything that you can do other than take the medicine or use the creams. I would rather have it there where it isn't too painful or visible to me.

I use hydrogen peroxide in a spray bottle to blast my lower area, it's really inexpensive and the results are great. I've also had success with DMSO cream, this I found online.

Still get really down about it as well but as time goes on you will end up feeling a little bit better. I have Zovirax cream and ointment. The cream is generally for cold sores (type I) but in my case I have type I orally and type I genitally as well so sometimes the cold sore creams work better down there too. It is strange. I also take l-lysine tablets that seem to help a lot and at GNC there is an l-lysine cream. It is almost like Vaseline looking but it is l-lysine and that seems to speed the healing process as well. I also have Valtrex pills that I take when I feel it coming on or if it has already come out.

I was just diagnosed with genital herpes and had my first outbreak just shy of two weeks ago. It was horrible and I ended up in the hospital with a catheter because I couldn't pee on my own. Now most of the lesions are gone and the last couple that are healing itch unbearably bad. Like I haven't been able to sleep through the night without waking up to itch and I can't sit still, etc.

Without having to go back to the doctor is there a way I can sooth the itching? and how long does this stage typically last?

Depends on if it is from yeast or just healing sores. I would try some Monistat at night and see if that helps you get thru. Did the doc prescribe any Valtrex or Zovirax?

This may sound extremely strange, but this advice was given to me nearly 40 years ago when I first contracted herpes. Mine shows up only on my lower back, so this isn't quite as painful as it might be for you. Cheap nail polish remover applied with a clean cotton ball will sting like heck for a couple of minutes, but it seems to kill the bugs on the surface and for me itching always stops! Good luck. You might try just a teeny bit to see if you can stand the stinging.

> No, no,no don't put fingernail polish remover in that area. The sores are healing. They will go away soon. Ask for Valtrex prevent more outbreaks. The first outbreak is the worst.

> I read that peeing in water, like a bath, helps a lot with not feeling the sting.

History

Herpes antiviral therapy began in the early 1960s with the experimental use of medication that interfered with viral replication called deoxyribonucleic acid (DNA) inhibitors. The original use was against normally fatal or disabilitating illness such as adult encephalitis,[83] keratitis,[84] in immunocompromised (transplant) patients,[85] or disseminated herpes zoster.[86] The original compounds used were 5-iodo-2'-deoxyuridine, AKA idoxuridine, IUdR, or(IDU) and 1-β-D-arabinofuranosylcytosine or ara-C,[87] later marketed under the name cytosar or cytorabine. The usage expanded to include topical treatment of herpes simplex,[88] zoster, and varicella.[89] Some trials combined different antivirals with differing results.[83] The introduction of 9-β-D-arabinofuranosyladenine, AKA ara-A or vidarabine, considerably less toxic than Ara-C, in the mid 1970s, heralded the way for the beginning of regular neonatal antiviral treatment.

Vidarabine was the first systemically administered antiviral medication with activity against HSV for which therapeutic efficacy outweighed toxicity for the management of life-threatening HSV disease. Intravenous vidarabine was licensed for use by the U.S. Food and Drug Administration (FDA) in 1977. Other experimental antivirals of that period included: Heparin[90], trifluorothymidine (TFT)[91], Ribivarin,[92] interferon,[93] Virazole,[94] and 5-methoxymethyl-2'-deoxyuridine (MMUdR).[95] The introduction of 9-(2-hydroxyethoxymethyl)guanine, AKA acyclovir, in the late 1970s[96] raised antiviral treatment another notch and led to vidarabine vs. acyclovir trials in the late 1980s.[97] The lower toxicity and ease of administration over vidarabine has led to acyclovir becoming the drug of choice for herpes treatment after it was licensed by the FDA in 1998.[98] Another advantage in the treatment of neonatal herpes included greater reductions in mortality and morbidity with increased dosages, something that did not occur when compared with increased dosages of vidarabine.[98] On the other side of the equation, acyclovir seems to inhibit antibody response and newborns on acyclovir antiviral treatment experienced a slower rise in antibody titer than those on vidarabine.[98]

Antiviral Medication

Antiviral medications used against herpes viruses work by interfering with viral replication, effectively slowing the replication rate of the virus and providing a greater opportunity for the immune response to intervene. All drugs in this class depend on the activity of the viral enzyme thymidine kinase to convert the drug sequentially from its prodrug form to monophosphate (with one phosphate group), diphosphate (with two phosphate groups), and finally to the triphosphate (with three phosphate groups) form which interferes with viral DNA replication.[99]

There are several prescription antiviral medications for controlling herpes simplex outbreaks, including acyclovir (Zovirax), valacyclovir (Valtrex), famciclovir (Famvir), and penciclovir. Acyclovir was the original, and prototypical, member of this drug class; it is now available in generic brands at a greatly reduced cost. Valacyclovir and famciclovir—prodrugs of acyclovir and penciclovir, respectively—have improved solubility in water and better bioavailability when taken orally.[99] Acyclovir is the recommended antiviral for suppressive therapy for use during the last months of pregnancy to prevent transmission of herpes simplex to the neonate in cases of maternal recurrent herpes.[100] The use of valacyclovir and famciclovir, while potentially improving treatment compliance and efficacy, are still undergoing safety evaluation in this context.

Several studies in humans and mice provide evidence that early treatment with famciclovir soon after the first infection with herpes can significantly lower the chance of future outbreaks of herpes. Early use of famciclovir has been shown to reduce the amount of latent virus in the neural ganglia.[101][102][103] A review of human subjects treated for five days with famciclovir 250 mg three times daily during their first herpes episode found that only 4.2 percent experienced a recurrence within six months after the first outbreak, a fivefold decrease compared to the 19 percent recurrence in acyclovir-treated patients.[104] Despite these promising results, early famciclovir treatment for herpes in this or similar dosage regimes has yet to find mainstream adoption. As a result, some doctors and patients have opted for off-label use. One suggested regime is famciclovir at 10–20 mg/kg per day for 5–10 days, with treatment to commence as soon as possible after the first herpes infection(not the first symptoms or outbreak), and the most effective time for initiating treatment to be five days or less after the first herpes infection. However, the window of opportunity for this treatment is only a few months after first infection with the virus, following this the potential effect on latency drops to zero.[105]

Antiviral medications are also available as topical creams for treating recurrent outbreaks on the lips, although their effectiveness is disputed.[106] Penciclovir cream has a 7–17 hour longer cellular half-life than acyclovir cream, increasing its effectiveness relative to acyclovir when topically applied.[107]

I was just diagnosed in April and since then have had about six outbreaks. I don't have a spleen so I have no immune system. The doctor put me on Acyclovir 400mg twice a day and that is not helping. Any advice would be greatly appreciated!

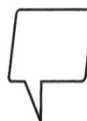

Your immune system is compromised by the absence of your spleen. Go back to your doctor and explain that the acyclovir is not helping. Possibly ask your doctor to prescribe a higher dose.

Web sites to find any vitamins/supplements that can help boost your immune system. Dr. Weil's Web site is pretty well known. Unfortunately, the first year of having herpes = lots of outbreaks.

Usually with time (crossing my fingers for you) the virus will calm down.

There is no question that oral acyclovir is a wonderful medication for relieving the pain and reducing the frequency of outbreaks of HSV-1 and 2. However, its effectiveness often leads sufferers to the mistaken conclusion that it also eliminates the risk of transmission when the sores are not present.

There is a substantial amount of medical evidence available on the Internet stating categorically that asymptomatic shedding can still take place in sufferers who are on constant medication with oral acyclovir. This can therefore increase the risk of transmission because the sufferer does not realize that they are in a shedding period.

There is a strong recommendation that it is better to take this drug IMMEDIATELY the first signs of an outbreak appear and for no longer than five days. That treatment is usually very effective and allows the sufferer to recognize and anticipate the frequency of outbreaks.

By employing good hygiene during the intervals between outbreaks, the risk of sexual transmission of the virus is then much more likely to be reduced or eliminated.

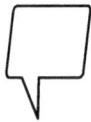

I always advise against the constant use of medication in circumstances where it is not necessary.

Just read the list of potential side-effects of acyclovir and you will see that this (and most other medicinal products) has the potential to do you harm. You might go for months or even years before your next outbreak so why subject your body to the risk of damage when it is not necessary?

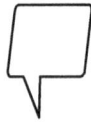

You're right, all meds do come with side effects.... even my birth control pills, asthma preventative and emergency inhaler come with side effects but I still take them every day and can't imagine not taking them until I needed them. I'll even take a pill to prevent a migraine if I know I'm going to be in the sun all day since I know sunlight triggers my migraines. I haven't had any side effects from acyclovir but have only been taking it for a month. Usually for me, if I am going to have any type of side effect it happens very quickly. But I'll definitely keep any eye out.

I'm not talking about the pills that you take once in a while to relieve or prevent an aggravating condition and I'm not talking about the long-term damaging treatments that improve the quality of life of a seriously ill sufferer, even though they may eventually cause death.

What concerns me is the long-term use of drugs that may gradually erode your internal organs without you being aware of it until too late - especially when their long-term use is of doubtful value. Furthermore, you have to consider the potential for viruses to develop resistance to a drug - meaning that, while it may work today, it might not work in ten years time.

Taking a pill every day because it may help to avoid the onset of an outbreak once a year makes no sense, particularly when the sufferer has plenty of time to recognize the warning signs and take the medication to stop the outbreak immediately. Side-effects are not necessarily evident to the user so, is it really worth the risk of long-term damage simply to avoid a couple of days of irritation?

Take a look around the Internet and you will see that I am not the only writer to advocate moderation in the use of anti-viral drugs.

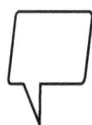

I have been taking acyclovir for YEARS. No problem. No problems with my blood work when I have it drawn. I have frequent outbreaks, so for me it is my choice to be on a daily suppressive.

I highly recommend going on a daily suppressive especially for the newly diagnosed. Your nerves/ emotions are on a roller coaster. It helps you differentiate what is an oncoming outbreak versus just nerves. If outbreaks have been calm to non-existent, try to go off the meds for a few months. I could not do that.

All medications have side effects. Each individual is different in what they experience. It is not a "blanket" this will harm you.

Everyone has freedom of choice - however, they should be aware of the risks.

Maybe by this time next year if I have not had any outbreaks, then I will consult with my gynecologist and see what's best, but for now I'm sticking to what my gynecologist advised me which is to take Acyclovir daily. Everyone is different but I have a high stress job and again, no time to wait or figure out if this is an actual outbreak...at least for now I know this is recent, I'm in a very committed

long-lasting relationship and already in the
routine of taking Acyclovir daily. My pharmacy
and gynecologist have covered the risks and in
their opinion, this med isn't life threatening to me.
However, if someone suffers from other diseases,
low immune system or anything else then their
doc may tell them Acyclovir isn't the right med
for them. Again, everyone is different. And every
doctor has their own opinion. And maybe even
each country has their own way of treating/
preventing this virus.

How long does an outbreak last for a woman?

That depends on several factors such as general
state of health, hygiene, neglect or treatment
and, if treated with acyclovir, at what point in an
outbreak that treatment is started.

*In a healthy woman, with good hygiene but no
medication it could be seven days or more but with
oral acyclovir taken at the start of an outbreak it
can be a day or two before the symptoms subside.*

Two days for me.

Topical Treatments

Docosanol is available as a cream for direct application to the affected area of skin. It prevents HSV from fusing to cell membranes, thus barring the entry of the virus into the skin. Docosanol was approved for use after clinical trials by the FDA in July 2000.[108] Docosanol is marketed by Avanir Pharmaceuticals under the name Abreva. It was the first over-the-counter antiviral drug approved for sale in the United States and Canada. Avanir Pharmaceuticals and GlaxoSmithKline Consumer Healthcare was the subject of a U.S. nationwide class-action suit in March, 2007 due to the misleading claim that it cut recovery times in half.[109]

Tromantadine is available as a gel that inhibits the entry and spread of the virus by altering the surface composition of skin cells and inhibiting release of viral genetic material. Zilactin is a topical analgesic barrier treatment, which forms a "shield" at the area of application to prevent a sore from increasing in size, and decrease viral spreading during the healing process.

Lipactin by Novartis is another over-the-counter topical gel which has been clinically shown to reduce symptoms and healing duration of a herpes simplex infection.

There is some limited research that has shown that tea tree oil may have topical anti-viral activity, especially with the herpes virus.[110]

Other Drugs

Cimetidine, a common component of heartburn medication, and probenecid have been shown to reduce the renal clearance of acyclovir.[111] These compounds also reduce the rate, but not the extent, at which valacyclovir is converted into acyclovir.

Limited evidence suggests that low dose aspirin (125 mg daily) might be beneficial in patients with recurrent HSV infections. Aspirin (acetylsalicylic acid) is an non-steroidal anti-inflammatory drug which reduces the level of prostaglandins—naturally occurring lipid compounds—that are essential in creating inflammation.[112] A recent study in animals showed inhibition of thermal (heat) stress induced viral shedding of HSV-1 in the eye by aspirin, and a possible benefit in reducing the frequency of recurrences.[113]

Another treatment is the use of petroleum jelly. Healing of cold sores is sped by barring water or saliva from reaching the sore.

Vaccines

The National Institutes of Health (NIH) in the United States is currently conducting phase III trials of Herpevac, a vaccine against HSV-2.[114] The vaccine has only been shown to be effective for women who have never been exposed to HSV-1. Overall, the vaccine is approximately 48% effective in preventing HSV-2 seropositivity and about 78% effective in preventing symptomatic HSV-2.[114] During initial trials, the vaccine did not exhibit any evidence of preventing HSV-2 in males.[114] Additionally, the vaccine only reduced the acquisition of HSV-2 and symptoms due to newly acquired HSV-2 among women who did not have HSV-2 infection at the time they got the vaccine.[114] Because about 20% of persons in the United States have HSV-2 infection, this further reduces the population for whom this vaccine might be appropriate.[114]

Researchers at the University of Florida have made a hammerhead ribozyme that targets and cleaves the mRNA of essential genes in HSV-1. The hammerhead which targets the mRNA of the UL20 gene greatly reduced the level of HSV-1 ocular infection in rabbits and reduced the viral yield in vivo.[115]

Natural Compounds

Many people seek benefits in natural products and dietary supplements for treatment of herpes

Certain dietary adjustments, dietary supplements, and alternative remedies are believed to be beneficial in the treatment of herpes, either alone, or in conjunction with prescribed antiviral therapy. There is currently insufficient scientific and clinical evidence to support the effective use of many of these compounds to treat herpes in humans.[116]

Lysine supplementation has been used for the prophylaxis and treatment of herpes simplex although doses smaller than 1 gram per day appear to be ineffective.[117][118][119]

Aloe Vera, available as a cream or gel, makes an affected area heal faster and may prevent recurrences.[120]

Lemon balm (Melissa officinalis) has antiviral activity against HSV-2 in cell culture and may reduce HSV symptoms in herpes infected people.[121][122][122]

Carrageenans—linear sulphated polysaccharides extracted from red seaweeds—have been shown to have antiviral effects in HSV-infected cells and in mice.[123][124]

There is conflicting evidence on a possible benefit from extracts from the plant Echinacea in treating oral[125], but not genital, herpes.[126]

Resveratrol, a compound naturally produced by plants and a component of red wine, prevents HSV replication in cultured cells and reduces cutaneous HSV lesion formation in mice. It is not considered potent enough to be an effective treatment on its own.[127][128]

Extracts from garlic have shown antiviral activity against HSV in cell culture experiments, although the extremely high concentrations of the extracts required to produce an antiviral effect was also toxic to the cells.[129]

The plant Prunella vulgaris, commonly known as selfheal, also prevents expression of both type 1 and type 2 herpes in cultured cells.[130]

Lactoferrin, a component of whey protein, has been shown to have a synergistic effect with acyclovir against HSV in vitro.[131]

Some dietary supplements have been suggested to positively treat herpes. These include vitamin C, vitamin A, vitamin E, and zinc.[132][133]

Butylated hydroxytoluene (BHT), commonly available as a food preservative, has been shown in cell culture and animal studies to inactivate herpes virus.[134][135] However, BHT has not been clinically tested and approved to treat herpes infections in humans.

Valtrex just keeps the healthy cells safe from the virus, so it doesn't spread from cell to cell. The other stuff, like camphophenic is just menthol and numbing stuff, which is just supposed to make it feel numb. You should try to vitamin section Lysine. It helps and is way cheaper than Valtrex.

There is also a lysine ointment that is almost like Vaseline that you can buy at GNC that you can put

on an actual sore. It is soothing and heals as well.
They have done studies on lysine that when put in
a dish with the herpes virus it was shown to attack
and kill off the virus. I take it frequently as well and
it does seem to work.

PSYCHOLOGICAL AND SOCIAL EFFECTS

Some people experience negative feelings related to the condition following diagnosis, particularly if they have acquired the genital form of the disease. Feelings can include depression, fear of rejection, feelings of isolation, fear of being found out, self-destructive feelings, and fear of masturbation.[136] These feelings usually lessen over time. Herpes support groups have been formed in the United States and the UK, providing information about herpes and running message forums and dating websites for sufferers.[137][138][139][140][141][142][143][144]

People with the herpes virus are often hesitant to divulge to other people, including friends and family, that they are infected. This is especially true of new or potential sexual partners that they consider casual.[145] A perceived reaction is sometimes taken into account before making a decision about whether to inform new partners and at what point in the relationship. Many people choose not to disclose their herpes status when they first begin dating someone, but wait until it later becomes clear that they are moving towards a sexual relationship. Other people disclose their herpes status upfront. Still others choose only to date other people who already have herpes.

I'm wondering how any of you in this situation explained it to someone new in your life? Did you wait until things got serious or explain it right from the beginning? How and what do you say? I really like this guy and I don't want to scare him away...but I feel dirty and contaminated and would completely understand if he did want to never speak to me again (Things are still new between us). Things are "heating up" between us and this is an entirely new situation to me.

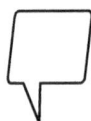

Were you diagnosed with high or low risk HPV?

I was diagnosed with low risk.

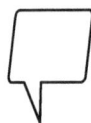

I had HPV for years and never told any of my partners. It is a virus that is transferrable but can go away, like it has in my case. Just do what you feel is right for you. Keep getting pap smears every six months.

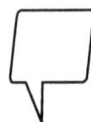

Now as far as genital herpes if you have that I feel it is very important to tell your partner up front before any sexual contact would take place. I got genital herpes 2 years ago from a man the first night we slept together, he took off the condom. He never told me he had this incurable disease until 6 months into the relationship when he had an outbreak. I stayed in the relationship because I felt that no other man would want me. We are on the outs now, and I'm at the point of dating again and I haven't slept with anyone new yet but, I believe in honesty upfront. The guy I just started talking to was very understanding and was comforting to me. He wanted to kill my ex though. I haven't had any outbreaks so far in two years but I do have this terrible but livable disease.

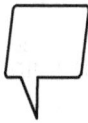

I would suggest you first coming out by telling him how common the disease is and letting him know how you got it how long you've had it and also let him know before even jumping to any conclusion of the relationship that he should get test also to be sure that he doesn't already have it...In males its harder to trace because they usually have limited to no outbreaks. Hopefully he's heard of HPV and let him know that it is an STD but you can get it even if you wear a condom because it's transmitted through skin to skin contact.

REFERENCES – HERPES SIMPLEX VIRUS

1. Ryan KJ, Ray CG (editors) (2004). Sherris Medical Microbiology (4th ed. ed.). McGraw Hill. pp. 555–62. ISBN 0838585299.

2. "Herpes simplex". DermNet NZ — New Zealand Dermatological Society. 2006-09-16. http://www.dermnetnz.org/viral/herpes-simplex.html. Retrieved on 2006-10-15.

3. Gupta R, Warren T, Wald A (2007). "Genital herpes". Lancet **370** (9605): 2127–37. doi:10.1016/S0140-6736(07)61908-4. PMID 18156035.

4. Kimberlin DW (2007). "Herpes simplex virus infections of the newborn". Semin. Perinatol. **31** (1): 19–25. doi:10.1053/j.semperi.2007.01.003. PMID 17317423.

5. Mettenleiter TC, Klupp BG, Granzow H (2006). "Herpesvirus assembly: a tale of two membranes". Curr. Opin. Microbiol. **9** (4): 423–9. doi:10.1016/j.mib.2006.06.013. PMID 16814597.

6. McGeoch DJ, Rixon FJ, Davison AJ (2006). "Topics in herpesvirus genomics and evolution". Virus Res. **117** (1): 90–104. doi:10.1016/j.virusres.2006.01.002. PMID 16490275.

7. Rajcáni J, Andrea V, Ingeborg R (2004). "Peculiarities of herpes simplex virus (HSV) transcription: an overview". Virus Genes **28** (3): 293–310. doi:10.1023/B:VIRU.0000025777.62826.92. PMID 15266111.

8. Search in UniProt Knowledgebase (Swiss-Prot and TrEMBL) for: HHV1

9. Matis J, Kúdelová M (2001). "Early shutoff of host protein synthesis in cells infected with herpes simplex viruses". Acta Virol. **45** (5-6): 269–77. PMID 12083325.

10. Wyrwicz LS, Ginalski K, Rychlewski L (2007). "HSV-1 UL45 encodes a carbohydrate binding C-type lectin protein". Cell Cycle **7** (2). PMID 18256535.

11. Vittone V, Diefenbach E, Triffett D, Douglas MW, Cunningham AL, Diefenbach RJ (2005). "Determination of interactions between tegument proteins of herpes simplex virus type 1". J. Virol. **79** (15): 9566–71. doi:10.1128/JVI.79.15.9566-9571.2005. PMID 16014918.

12. Subramanian RP, Geraghty RJ (2007). "Herpes simplex virus type 1 mediates fusion through a hemifusion intermediate by sequential activity of glycoproteins D, H, L, and B". Proc. Natl. Acad. Sci. U.S.A. **104** (8): 2903–8. doi:10.1073/pnas.0608374104. PMID 17299053.

13. Cardone G, Winkler DC, Trus BL, Cheng N, Heuser JE, Newcomb WW, Brown JC, Steven AC (May 2007). "Visualization of the herpes simplex virus portal in situ by cryo-electron tomography". Virology **361** (2): 426–34. doi:10.1016/j.virol.2006.10.047. PMID 17188319.

14. Trus BL, Cheng N, Newcomb WW, Homa FL, Brown JC, Steven AC (November 2004). "Structure and polymorphism of the UL6 portal protein of herpes simplex virus type 1". *Journal of Virology* **78** (22): 12668–71. doi:10.1128/JVI.78.22.12668-12671.2004. PMID 15507654.(Article: [1])

15. Nellissery JK, Szczepaniak R, Lamberti C, Weller SK (2007-06-20). "A putative leucine zipper within the HSV-1 UL6 protein is required for portal ring formation". Journal Virology. PMID 17581990.

16. Newcomb WW, Booy FP, Brown JC (2007). "Uncoating the herpes simplex virus genome". *J. Mol. Biol.* **370** (4): 633–42. doi:10.1016/j.jmb.2007.05.023. PMID 17540405.

17. Adang LA, Parsons CH, Kedes DH (2006). "Asynchronous progression through the lytic cascade and variations in intracellular viral loads revealed by high-throughput single-cell analysis of Kaposi's sarcoma-associated herpesvirus infection". *J. Virol.* **80** (20): 10073–82. doi:10.1128/JVI.01156-06. PMID 17005685.

18. Taddeo B, Roizman B (2006). "The virion host shutoff protein (UL41) of herpes simplex virus 1 is an endoribonuclease with a substrate specificity similar to that of RNase A". *J. Virol.* **80** (18): 9341–5. doi:10.1128/JVI.01008-06. PMID 16940547.

19. Skepper JN, Whiteley A, Browne H, Minson A (June 2001). "Herpes simplex virus nucleocapsids mature to progeny virions by an envelopment --> deenvelopment --> reenvelopment pathway". *J. Virol.* **75** (12): 5697–702. doi:10.1128/JVI.75.12.5697-5702.2001. PMID 11356979.

20. Granzow H, Klupp BG, Fuchs W, Veits J, Osterrieder N, Mettenleiter TC (April 2001). "Egress of alphaherpesviruses: comparative ultrastructural study". *J. Virol.* **75** (8): 3675–84. doi:10.1128/JVI.75.8.3675-3684.2001. PMID 11264357.

21. Pinnoji RC, Bedadala GR, George B, Holland TC, Hill JM, Hsia SC (2007). "Repressor element-1 silencing transcription factor/neuronal restrictive silencer factor (REST/NRSF) can regulate HSV-1 immediate-early transcription via histone modification". *Virol. J.* **4**: 56. doi:10.1186/1743-422X-4-56. PMID 17555596.

22. Pinnoji RC, Bedadala GR, George B, Holland TC, Hill JM, Hsia SC (2007). "Repressor element-1 silencing transcription factor/neuronal restrictive silencer factor (REST/NRSF) can regulate HSV-1 immediate-early transcription via histone modification". *Virol. J.* **4**: 56. doi:10.1186/1743-422X-4-56. PMID 17555596.

23. Bedadala GR, Pinnoji RC, Hsia SC (2007). "Early growth response gene 1 (Egr-1) regulates HSV-1 ICP4 and ICP22 gene expression". *Cell Res.* **17** (6): 546–55. doi:10.1038/cr.2007.44. PMID 17502875.

24. Roizman B, Gu H, Mandel G (2005). "The first 30 minutes in the life of a virus: unREST in the nucleus". *Cell Cycle* **4** (8): 1019–21. PMID 16082207.

25. http://www.freepatentsonline.com/EP1021223.html. See : Description - Background of the invention.

26. http://www.google.com/patents?id=E8AoAAAAEBAJ&dq=US+5500009

27. Middleton PJ, Peteric M, Kozak M, Rewcastle NB, McLachlan DR. (1980). "Herpes simplex viral genome and senile and presenile dementias of Alzheimer and Pick.". *Lancet* **315:** 1038. doi:10.1016/S0140-6736(80)91490-7.

28. Dobson, C.B.; Itzhaki, R.F. (1999). "Herpes simplex virus type 1 and Alzheimer's disease.". *Neurobiol Aging* **20** (4): 457–65. doi:10.1016/S0197-4580(99)00055-X. http://www.ncbi.nlm.nih.gov/sites/entrez?db=pubmed&uid =10604441&cmd=showdetailview&indexed=google. Retrieved on 2008-03-15.

29. Pyles, R.B. (2001). "The association of herpes simplex virus and Alzheimer's disease: a potential synthesis of genetic and environmental factors" (PDF). *Herpes* **8** (3): 64–68. http://www.ihmf.com/journal/download/ 83pyles(64)vol864.pdf. Retrieved on 2008-03-15.

30. Itzhaki, R.F.; Lin, W.R.; Shang, D.; Wilcock, G.K.; Faragher, B.; Jamieson, G.A. (1997). "Herpes simplex virus type 1 in brain and risk of Alzheimer's disease.". *Lancet* **349** (9047): 241–4. doi:10.1016/S0140-6736(96)10149-5. http://www.ncbi. nlm.nih.gov/sites/entrez?db=pubmed&uid=97167222&cmd=showdetailview &indexed=google. Retrieved on 2008-03-15.

31. Wozniak, M.A; Mee, A.P; Itzhaki, R.F (2008). "Herpes simplex virus type 1 DNA is located within Alzheimer's disease amyloid plaques.". *The Journal of Pathology* **217** (1): 131–138. doi:10.1002/path.2449. http://www3.interscience. wiley.com/journal/121411445/abstract. Retrieved on 2008-09-05.

REFERENCES: HERPES SIMPLEX 1 & 2

1. Dickerson FB, Boronow JJ, Stallings C, et al (March 2004). "Infection with herpes simplex virus type 1 is associated with cognitive deficits in bipolar disorder". Biol. Psychiatry **55** (6): 588–93. doi:10.1016/j.biopsych.2003.10.008. PMID 15013827.

2. Itzhaki RF, Lin WR, Shang D, Wilcock GK, Faragher B, Jamieson GA (January 1997). "Herpes simplex virus type 1 in brain and risk of Alzheimer's disease". Lancet **349** (9047): 241–4. doi:10.1016/S0140-6736(96)10149-5. PMID 9014911.

3. Gupta R, Warren T, Wald A (December 2007). "Genital herpes". Lancet **370** (9605): 2127–37. doi:10.1016/S0140-6736(07)61908-4. PMID 18156035. http://linkinghub.elsevier.com/retrieve/pii/S0140-6736(07)61908-4.

4. Brown ZA, Selke S, Zeh J, et al (August 1997). "The acquisition of herpes simplex virus during pregnancy". N Engl J Med. **337** (8): 509–15. doi:10.1056/NEJM199708213370801. PMID 9262493. http://content.nejm.org/cgi/content/full/337/8/509.

5. Fleming, Thomas R. (2008). "Linear erosive Herpes Simplex Virus infection in immunocompromised patients: the "Knife-Cut Sign"". Clin Infect Dis **47**: 1440–1441. doi:10.1086/591390.

6. Takasu T, Furuta Y, Sato KC, Fukuda S, Inuyama Y, Nagashima K (1992). "Detection of latent herpes simplex virus DNA and RNA in human geniculate ganglia by the polymerase chain reaction". Acta Otolaryngol. **112** (6): 1004–11. doi:10.3109/00016489209137502. PMID 1336296.

7. Sugita T, Murakami S, Yanagihara N, Fujiwara Y, Hirata Y, Kurata T (1995). "Facial nerve paralysis induced by herpes simplex virus in mice: an animal model of acute and transient facial paralysis". Ann. Otol. Rhinol. Laryngol. **104** (7): 574–81. PMID 7598372.

8. Lazarini PR, Vianna MF, Alcantara MP, Scalia RA, Caiaffa Filho HH (2006). "Herpes simplex virus in the saliva of peripheral Bell's palsy patients" (in Portuguese). Rev Bras Otorrinolaringol (Engl Ed) **72** (1): 7–11. PMID 16917546.

9. Linder T, Bossart W, Bodmer D (2005). "Bell's palsy and Herpes simplex virus: fact or mystery?". Otol. Neurotol. **26** (1): 109–13. doi:10.1097/00129492-200501000-00020. PMID 15699730.

10. Kanerva M, Mannonen L, Piiparinen H, Peltomaa M, Vaheri A, Pitkäranta A (2007). "Search for Herpesviruses in cerebrospinal fluid of facial palsy patients by PCR". Acta Otolaryngol. **127** (7): 775–9. doi:10.1080/00016480601011444. PMID 17573575.

11. Stjernquist-Desatnik A, Skoog E, Aurelius E (2006). "Detection of herpes simplex and varicella-zoster viruses in patients with Bell's palsy by the polymerase chain reaction technique". Ann. Otol. Rhinol. Laryngol. **115** (4): 306–11. PMID 16676828.

12. Tiemstra JD, Khatkhate N (2007). "Bell's palsy: diagnosis and management". *Am Fam Physician* **76** (7): 997–1002. PMID 17956069.

13. Middleton PJ, Peteric M, Kozak M, Rewcastle NB, McLachlan DR. (1980). "Herpes simplex viral genome and senile and presenile dementias of Alzheimer and Pick.". *Lancet* **315**: 1038. doi:10.1016/S0140-6736(80)91490-7.

14. Dobson CB, Itzhaki RF (1999). "Herpes simplex virus type 1 and Alzheimer's disease". *Neurobiol. Aging* **20** (4): 457–65. doi:10.1016/S0197-4580(99)00055-X. PMID 10604441. http://linkinghub.elsevier.com/retrieve/pii/S0197-4580(99)00055-X.

15. Pyles RB (November 2001). "The association of herpes simplex virus and Alzheimer's disease: a potential synthesis of genetic and environmental factors". *Herpes* **8** (3): 64–8. PMID 11867022. http://www.ihmf.com/journal/download/83pyles(64)vol864.pdf.

16. Itzhaki RF, Lin WR, Shang D, Wilcock GK, Faragher B, Jamieson GA (January 1997). "Herpes simplex virus type 1 in brain and risk of Alzheimer's disease". *Lancet* **349** (9047): 241–4. doi:10.1016/S0140-6736(96)10149-5. PMID 9014911.

17. Wozniak MA, Mee AP, Itzhaki RF (January 2009). "Herpes simplex virus type 1 DNA is located within Alzheimer's disease amyloid plaques". *J Pathol.* **217** (1): 131–8. doi:10.1002/path.2449. PMID 18973185. http://www3.interscience.wiley.com/journal/121411445/abstract.

18. Stumpf MP, Laidlaw Z, Jansen VA (2002). "Herpes viruses hedge their bets". *Proc. Natl. Acad. Sci. U.S.A.* **99** (23): 15234–7. doi:10.1073/pnas.232546899. PMID 12409612. http://www.pnas.org/content/99/23/15234.

19. Sainz B, Loutsch JM, Marquart ME, Hill JM (2001). "Stress-associated immunomodulation and herpes simplex virus infections". *Med. Hypotheses* **56** (3): 348–56. doi:10.1054/mehy.2000.1219. PMID 11359358.

20. http://www.sciencenews.org/view/generic/id/42223/title/How_herpes_re-rears_its_ugly_head_

21. Myśliwska J, Trzonkowski P, Bryl E, Lukaszuk K, Myśliwski A (2000). "Lower interleukin-2 and higher serum tumor necrosis factor-a levels are associated with perimenstrual, recurrent, facial Herpes simplex infection in young women". *Eur. Cytokine Netw.* **11** (3): 397–406. PMID 11022124.

22. Segal AL, Katcher AH, Brightman VJ, Miller MF (1974). "Recurrent herpes labialis, recurrent aphthous ulcers, and the menstrual cycle". *J. Dent. Res.* **53** (4): 797–803. PMID 4526372.

23. Chambers A, Perry M (2008). "Salivary mediated autoinoculation of herpes simplex virus on the face in the absence of "cold sores," after trauma". *J. Oral Maxillofac. Surg.* **66** (1): 136–8. doi:10.1016/j.joms.2006.07.019. PMID 18083428.

24. Perna JJ, Mannix ML, Rooney JF, Notkins AL, Straus SE (1987). "Reactivation of latent herpes simplex virus infection by ultraviolet light: a human model". *J. Am. Acad. Dermatol.* **17** (3): 473–8. doi:10.1016/S0190-9622(87)70232-1. PMID 2821086.

25. Rooney JF, Straus SE, Mannix ML, *et al* (1992). "UV light-induced reactivation of herpes simplex virus type 2 and prevention by acyclovir". *J. Infect. Dis.* **166** (3): 500–6. PMID 1323616.

26. Oakley C, Epstein JB, Sherlock CH (1997). "Reactivation of oral herpes simplex virus: implications for clinical management of herpes simplex virus recurrence during radiotherapy". *Oral Surg Oral Med Oral Pathol Oral Radiol Endod* **84** (3): 272–8. doi:10.1016/S1079-2104(97)90342-5. PMID 9377190.

27. Ichihashi M, Nagai H, Matsunaga K (2004). "Sunlight is an important causative factor of recurrent herpes simplex". *Cutis* **74** (5 Suppl): 14–8. PMID 15603217.

28. Martinez V, Caumes E, Chosidow O (2008). "Treatment to prevent recurrent genital herpes". *Curr Opin Infect Dis* **21** (1): 42–48. doi:10.1097/QCO.0b013e3282f3d9d3. PMID 18192785.

29. "AHMF: Preventing Sexual Transmission of Genital herpes". http://www.ahmf.com.au/health_professionals/guidelines/preventing_gh_transmission.htm. Retrieved on 2008-02-24.

30. Leone P (2005). "Reducing the risk of transmitting genital herpes: advances in understanding and therapy". *Curr Med Res Opin* **21** (10): 1577–82. doi:10.1185/030079905X61901. PMID 16238897.

31. Kim H, Meier A, Huang M, Kuntz S, Selke S, Celum C, Corey L, Wald A (2006). "Oral herpes simplex virus type 2 reactivation in HIV-positive and -negative men.". *J Infect Dis* **194** (4): 420–7. doi:10.1086/505879. PMID 16845624.

32. Mertz, G.J. (1993). "Epidemiology of genital herpes infections.". *Infect Dis Clin North Am* **7** (4): 825–39. PMID 8106731.

33. Wald A, Langenberg AG, Link K, Izu AE, Ashley R, Warren T, Tyring S, Douglas JM Jr, Corey L. (2001). "Effect of condoms on reducing the transmission of herpes simplex virus type 2 from men to women". *JAMA* **285** (24): 3100–3106. doi:10.1001/jama.285.24.3100. PMID 11427138. http://jama.ama-assn.org/cgi/content/full/285/24/3100.

34. Casper C, Wald A. (2002). "Condom use and the prevention of genital herpes acquisition," (PDF). *Herpes* **9** (1): 10–14. PMID 11916494. http://www.ihmf.org/journal/download/91casper(10)vol910.pdf.

35. de Visser RO, Smith AM, Rissel CE, Richters J, Grulich AE. (2003). "Sex in Australia: safer sex and condom use among a representative sample of adults". *Aust. N. Z. J. Public Health.* **27** (2): 223–229. doi:10.1111/j.1467-842X.2003.tb00812.x. PMID 14696715.

36. Seppa, Nathan (2005-01-05). "One-Two Punch: Vaccine fights herpes with antibodies, T cells" (in English). Science News. pp. 5. http://www.sciencenews.org/articles/20050101/fob6.asp. Retrieved on 2007-03-29.

37. Carla K. Johnson (August 23, 2006). "Percentage of people with herpes drops". Associated Press. http://www.newsobserver.com/150/story/477928.html.

38. Kulhanjian JA, Soroush V, Au DS, et al (02 April 1992). "Identification of women at unsuspected risk of primary infection with herpes simplex virus type 2 during pregnancy". N. Engl. J. Med. **326** (14): 916–20. PMID 1311799. http://content.nejm.org/cgi/content/abstract/326/14/916.

39. Corey L, Wald A, Patel R, et al (January 2004). "Once-daily valacyclovir to reduce the risk of transmission of genital herpes". N Engl J Med. **350** (1): 11–20. doi:10.1056/NEJMoa035144. PMID 14702423. http://content.nejm.org/cgi/reprint/350/1/11.pdf.

40. Wald A, Langenberg AG, Krantz E, et al (November 2005). "The relationship between condom use and herpes simplex virus acquisition". Ann Intern Med. **143** (10): 707–13. PMID 16287791. http://www.annals.org/cgi/reprint/143/10/707.

41. Template:Ref journal

42. Brown ZA, Wald A, Morrow RA, Selke S, Zeh J, Corey L (2003). "Effect of serologic status and cesarean delivery on transmission rates of herpes simplex virus from mother to infant". JAMA **289:** 203–209. doi:10.1001/jama.289.2.203. PMID 12517231.

43. Brown ZA, Benedetti J, Ashley R et al. (1991). "Neonatal herpes simplex virus infection in relation to asymptomatic maternal infection at the time of labor". N Engl J Med **324:** 1247.

44. Whitley RJ, Kimberlin DW, Roizman B (1998). "Herpes simplex viruses". Clin Infect Dis **26** (3): 541–53. doi:10.1086/514600. PMID 9524821. http://www.journals.uchicago.edu/doi/pdf/10.1086/514600.

45. Brown ZA, Benedetti J, Ashley R, et al (May 1991). "Neonatal herpes simplex virus infection in relation to asymptomatic maternal infection at the time of labor". N. Engl. J. Med. **324** (18): 1247–52. PMID 1849612.

46. Sobngwi-Tambekou J, Taljaard D, Lissouba P, et al. (2009). "Effect of HSV-2 Serostatus on Acquisition of HIV by Young Men: Results of a Longitudinal Study in Orange Farm, South Africa". J Infect Dis **199:** 958–964. doi:10.1086/597208.

47. Koelle DM, Corey L (2008). "Herpes Simplex: Insights on Pathogenesis and Possible Vaccines". Annu Rev Med **59:** 381–395. doi:10.1146/annurev.med.59.061606.095540. PMID 18186706.

48. Fatahzadeh M, Schwartz RA (2007). "Human herpes simplex virus infections: epidemiology, pathogenesis, symptomatology, diagnosis, and management". *J. Am. Acad. Dermatol.* **57** (5): 737–63; quiz 764–6. doi:10.1016/j.jaad.2007.06.027. PMID 17939933.

49. Handsfield HH (2000). "Public Health Strategies to Prevent Genital Herpes: Where Do We Stand?". *Curr Infect Dis Rep* **2** (1): 25–30. doi:10.1007/s11908-000-0084-y. PMID 11095834.

50. Smith JS, Robinson NJ (2002). "Age-specific prevalence of infection with herpes simplex virus types 2 and 1: a global review". *J. Infect. Dis.* **186 Suppl 1:** S3–28. doi:10.1086/343739. PMID 12353183. http://www.journals.uchicago.edu/doi/full/10.1086/343739.

51. Patnaik P, Herrero R, Morrow RA, *et al* (2007). "Type-specific seroprevalence of herpes simplex virus type 2 and associated risk factors in middle-aged women from 6 countries: the IARC multicentric study". *Sex Transm Dis* **34** (12): 1019–24. PMID 18080353. http://www.stdjournal.com/pt/re/std/abstract.00007435-200712000-00016.htm.

52. Shin HS, Park JJ, Chu C, *et al* (2007). "Herpes simplex virus type 2 seroprevalence in Korea: rapid increase of HSV-2 seroprevalence in the 30s in the southern part". *J. Korean Med. Sci.* **22** (6): 957–62. doi:10.3346/jkms.2007.22.6.957. PMID 18162706.

53. Pebody RG, Andrews N, Brown D, *et al* (2004). "The seroepidemiology of herpes simplex virus type 1 and 2 in Europe". *Sex Transm Infect* **80** (3): 185–91. doi:10.1136/sti.2003.005850. PMID 15170000. http://sti.bmj.com/cgi/content/abstract/80/3/185.

54. Mertz GJ, Rosenthal SL, Stanberry LR (October 2003). "Is herpes simplex virus type 1 (HSV-1) now more common than HSV-2 in first episodes of genital herpes?". *Sex Transm Dis* **30** (10): 801–2. doi:10.1097/01.OLQ.0000093080.55201.D1. PMID 14520182. http://meta.wkhealth.com/pt/pt-core/template-journal/lwwgateway/media/landingpage.htm?issn=0148-5717&volume=30&issue=10&spage=801.

55. Roberts CM, Pfister JR, Spear SJ (2003). "Increasing proportion of herpes simplex virus type 1 as a cause of genital herpes infection in college students" (PDF). *Sex Transm Dis* **30** (10): 797–800. doi:10.1097/01.OLQ.0000092387.58746.C7. PMID 14520181. http://www.stdjournal.com/pt/re/std/pdfhandler.00007435-200310000-00012.pdf.

56. Malkin JE (2004). "Epidemiology of genital herpes simplex virus infection in developed countries" (PDF). *Herpes* **11 Suppl 1:** 2A–23A. PMID 15115626. http://www.ihmf.org/journal/download/11Malkin(2A)sup12A.pdf.

57. "Herpes simplex" (in English) (HTML). University of Maryland Medical Center. http://www.umm.edu/patiented/articles/who_gets_herpes_simplex_virus_000052_4.htm. Retrieved on 2007-09-03.

58. "LEARN ABOUT HERPES > Fast Facts" (in English) (HTML). ASHA Herpes Resource Center. http://www.ashastd.org/herpes/herpes_learn.cfm. Retrieved on 2007-09-03.

59. "STD Facts - Genital Herpes" (in English) (HTML). Centers for Disease Control and Prevention. http://www.cdc.gov/std/Herpes/STDFact-Herpes.htm. Retrieved on 2007-09-03.

60. "Herpes" (in English) (HTML). Stanford University Sexual Health Peer Resource Center. http://www.stanford.edu/group/SHPRC/ch4_her.html. Retrieved on 2007-09-03.

61. Howard M, Sellors JW, Jang D, et al (January 2003). "Regional distribution of antibodies to herpes simplex virus type 1 (HSV-1) and HSV-2 in men and women in Ontario, Canada". *J Clin Microbiol.* **41** (1): 84–9. doi:10.1128/JCM.41.1.84-89.2003. PMID 12517830. PMC: 149555. http://jcm.asm.org/cgi/pmidlookup?view=long&pmid=12517830.

62. Patrick DM, Dawar M, Cook DA, Krajden M, Ng HC, Rekart ML (July 2001). "Antenatal seroprevalence of herpes simplex virus type 2 (HSV-2) in Canadian women: HSV-2 prevalence increases throughout the reproductive years". *Sex Transm Dis* **28** (7): 424–8. doi:10.1097/00007435-200107000-00011. PMID 11460028. http://www.stdjournal.com/pt/re/std/fulltext.00007435-200107000-00011.htm.

63. Singh AE, Romanowski B, Wong T, et al (February 2005). "Herpes simplex virus seroprevalence and risk factors in 2 Canadian sexually transmitted disease clinics". *Sex Transm Dis* **32** (2): 95–100. doi:10.1097/01.olq.0000151415.78210.85. PMID 15668615. http://www.stdjournal.com/pt/re/std/fulltext.00007435-200502000-00006.htm.

64. Forward KR, Lee SH (March 2003). "Predominance of herpes simplex virus type 1 from patients with genital herpes in Nova Scotia". *Can J Infect Dis* **14** (2): 94–6. PMID 18159431.

65. Weiss H (2004). "Epidemiology of herpes simplex virus type 2 infection in the developing world". *Herpes* **11 Suppl 1:** 24A–35A. PMID 15115627.

66. Loutfy SA, Alam El-Din HM, Ibrahim MF, Hafez MM (2006). "Seroprevalence of herpes simplex virus types 1 and 2, Epstein-Barr virus, and cytomegalovirus in children with acute lymphoblastic leukemia in Egypt Kundi". *Saudi Med J* **27** (8): 1139–45. PMID 16883441.

67. Meguenni S, Djenaoui T, Bendib A, et al (1989). "Herpes simplex virus infections in Algiers" (in French). *Arch Inst Pasteur Alger* **57:** 61–72. PMID 2562258.

68. Smith JS, Herrero R, Muñoz N, et al (2001). "Prevalence and risk factors for herpes simplex virus type 2 infection among middle-age women in Brazil and the Philippines". *Sex Transm Dis* **28** (4): 187–94. doi:10.1097/00007435-200104000-00001. PMID 11318248. http://www.stdjournal.com/pt/re/std/fulltext.00007435-200104000-00001.htm.

69. Kaur R, Gupta N, Baveja UK (2005). "Seroprevalence of HSV1 and HSV2 infections in family planning clinic attenders". *J Commun Dis* **37** (4): 307–9. PMID 17278662.

70. Dolar N, Serdaroglu S, Yilmaz G, Ergin S (2006). "Seroprevalence of herpes simplex virus type 1 and type 2 in Turkey". *J Eur Acad Dermatol Venereol* **20** (10): 1232–6. doi:10.1111/j.1468-3083.2006.01766.x. PMID 17062037.

71. Abuharfeil N, Meqdam MM (2000). "Seroepidemiologic study of herpes simplex virus type 2 and cytomegalovirus among young adults in northern Jordan". *New Microbiol.* **23** (3): 235–9. PMID 10939038.

72. Davidovici BB, Grotto I, Balicer RD, Robinson NJ, Cohen D (November 2006). "Decline in the prevalence of antibodies to herpes simplex virus types 1 and 2 among Israeli young adults between 1984 and 2002" (PDF). *Sex Transm Dis* **33** (11): 641–5. doi:10.1097/01.olq.0000216068.01028.38. PMID 16614586. http://www.stdjournal.com/pt/re/std/pdfhandler.00007435-200611000-00001.pdf.

73. Davidovici BB, Green M, Marouni MJ, Bassal R, Pimenta JM, Cohen D (2006). "Seroprevalence of herpes simplex virus 1 and 2 and correlates of infection in Israel". *J. Infect.* **52** (5): 367–73. doi:10.1016/j.jinf.2005.08.005. PMID 16213591.

74. Dan M, Sadan O., Glezerman M, Raveh D, Samra Z (2003). "Prevalence and risk factors for herpes simplex virus type 2 infection among pregnant women in Israel" (PDF). *Sex Transm Dis* **30(11):** 835–8. PMID 14603091. http://www.stdjournal.com/pt/re/std/pdfhandler.00007435-200311000-00007.pdf.

75. Feldman PA, Steinberg J, Madeb R, *et al* (September 2003). "Herpes simplex virus type 2 seropositivity in a sexually transmitted disease clinic in Israel" (PDF). *Isr. Med. Assoc. J.* **5** (9): 626–8. PMID 14509150. http://www.ima.org.il/imaj/ar03sep-5.pdf.

76. Samra Z, Scherf E, Dan M (2003). "Herpes simplex virus type 1 is the prevailing cause of genital herpes in the Tel Aviv area, Israel". *Sex Transm Dis* **30** (10): 794–6. doi:10.1097/01.OLQ.0000079517.04451.79. PMID 14520180. http://www.stdjournal.com/pt/re/std/fulltext.00007435-200310000-00011.htm.

77. Ibrahim AI, Kouwatli KM, Obeid MT (2000). "Frequency of herpes simplex virus in Syria based on type-specific serological assay". *Saudi Med J* **21** (4): 355–60. PMID 11533818.

78. Cunningham AL, Taylor R, Taylor J, Marks C, Shaw J, Mindel A (2006). "Prevalence of infection with herpes simplex virus types 1 and 2 in Australia: a nationwide population based survey". *Sex Transm Infect* **82** (2): 164–8. doi:10.1136/sti.2005.016899. PMID 16581748. http://sti.bmj.com/cgi/content/abstract/82/2/164.

79. Haddow LJ, Dave B, Mindel A, *et al* (2006). "Increase in rates of herpes simplex virus type 1 as a cause of anogenital herpes in western Sydney, Australia, between 1979 and 2003". *Sex Transm Infect* **82** (3): 255–9. doi:10.1136/sti.2005.018176. PMID 16731681. http://sti.bmj.com/cgi/content/abstract/82/3/255.

80. Lyttle PH (1994). "Surveillance report: disease trends at New Zealand sexually transmitted disease clinics 1977–1993". *Genitourin Med* **70** (5): 329–35. PMID 8001945.

81. "Local anesthetic creams". *BMJ* **297** (6661): 1468. 1988. PMID 3147021.

82. Kaminester LH, Pariser RJ, Pariser DM, *et al* (1999). "A double-blind, placebo-controlled study of topical tetracaine in the treatment of herpes labialis". *J. Am. Acad. Derm* **41** (6): 996–1001. doi:10.1016/S0190-9622(99)70260-4. PMID 10570387.

83. how AW, Roland A, Fiala M, *et al* (March 1973). "Cytosine arabinoside therapy for herpes simplex encephalitis--clinical experience with six patients". *Antimicrob. Agents Chemother.* **3** (3): 412–7. PMID 4790599. PMC: 444424. http://aac.asm.org/cgi/pmidlookup?view=long&pmid=4790599.

84. Kaufman HE, Howard GM (August 1962). "Therapy of experimental herpes simplex keratitis". *Invest Ophthalmol* **1**: 561–4. PMID 14454441. http://www.iovs.org/cgi/pmidlookup?view=long&pmid=14454441.

85. Ch'ien LT, Whitley RJ, Alford CA, Galasso GJ (June 1976). "Adenine arabinoside for therapy of herpes zoster in immunosuppressed patients: preliminary results of a collaborative study". *J. Infect. Dis.* **133 Suppl:** A184–91. PMID 180198.

86. McKelvey EM, Kwaan HC (November 1969). "Cytosine arabinoside therapy for disseminated herpes zoster in a patient with IgG pyroglobulinemia". *Blood* **34** (5): 706–11. PMID 5352659. http://www.bloodjournal.org/cgi/pmidlookup?view=long&pmid=5352659.

87. Fiala M, Chow A, Guze LB (April 1972). "Susceptibility of herpesviruses to cytosine arabinoside: standardization of susceptibility test procedure and relative resistance of herpes simplex type 2 strains". *Antimicrob. Agents Chemother.* **1** (4): 354–7. PMID 4364937. PMC: 444221. http://aac.asm.org/cgi/pmidlookup?view=long&pmid=4364937.

88. Allen LB, Hintz OJ, Wolf SM, *et al* (June 1976). "Effect of 9-beta-D-arabinofuranosylhypoxanthine 5'-monophosphate on genital lesions and encephalitis induced by Herpesvirus hominis type 2 in female mice". *J. Infect. Dis.* **133 Suppl:** A178–83. PMID 6598.

89. Juel-Jensen BE (March 1970). "Varicella and cytosine arabinoside". *Lancet* **1** (7646): 572. doi:10.1016/S0140-6736(70)90815-9. PMID 4190397.

90. Nahmias AJ, Kibrick S (May 1964). "Inhibitory effect of heparin on herpes simplex virus". *J. Bacteriol.* **87** (5): 1060–6. PMID 4289440. PMC: 277146. http://jb.asm.org/cgi/pmidlookup?view=long&pmid=4289440.

91. Allen LB, Sidwell RW (September 1972). "Target-organ treatment of neurotropic virus diseases: efficacy as a chemotherapy tool and comparison of activity of adenine arabinoside, cytosine arabinoside, idoxuridine, and trifluorothymidine". *Antimicrob. Agents Chemother.* **2** (3): 229–33. PMID 4790562. PMC: 444296. http://aac.asm.org/cgi/pmidlookup?view=long&pmid=4790562.

92. Allen LB, Wolf SM, Hintz CJ, Huffman JH, Sidwell RW (March 1977). "Effect of ribavirin on Type 2 Herpesvirus hominis (HVH/2) in vitro and in vivo". *Ann. N. Y. Acad. Sci.* **284:** 247–53. doi:10.1111/j.1749-6632.1977.tb21957.x. PMID 212976.

93. Allen LB, Cochran KW (November 1972). "Target-organ treatment of neurotropic virus disease with interferon inducers". *Infect. Immun.* **6** (5): 819–23. PMID 4404669. PMC: 422616. http://iai.asm.org/cgi/pmidlookup?view=long&pmid=4404669.

94. Sidwell RW, Huffman JH, Khare GP, Allen LB, Witkowski JT, Robins RK (August 1972). "Broad-spectrum antiviral activity of Virazole: 1-beta-D-ribofuranosyl-1,2,4-triazole-3-carboxamide". *Science (journal)* **177** (50): 705–6. PMID 4340949. http://www.sciencemag.org/cgi/pmidlookup?view=long&pmid=4340949.

95. Babiuk LA, Meldrum B, Gupta VS, Rouse BT (December 1975). "Comparison of the antiviral effects of 5-methoxymethyl-deoxyuridine with 5-iododeoxyuridine, cytosine arabinoside, and adenine arabinoside". Antimicrob. *Agents Chemother.* **8** (6): 643–50. PMID 1239978. PMC: 429441. http://aac.asm.org/cgi/pmidlookup?view=long&pmid=1239978.

96. O'Meara A, Deasy PF, Hillary IB, Bridgen WD (December 1979). "Acyclovir for treatment of mucocutaneous herpes infection in a child with leukaemia". *Lancet* **2** (8153): 1196. doi:10.1016/S0140-6736(79)92428-0. PMID 91931.

97. Whitley R, Arvin A, Prober C, *et al* (February 1991). "A controlled trial comparing vidarabine with acyclovir in neonatal herpes simplex virus infection. Infectious Diseases Collaborative Antiviral Study Group". *N. Engl. J. Med.* **324** (7): 444–9. PMID 1988829. http://content.nejm.org/cgi/content/abstract/324/7/444.

98. Kimberlin DW, Lin CY, Jacobs RF, *et al* (August 2001). "Safety and efficacy of high-dose intravenous acyclovir in the management of neonatal herpes simplex virus infections". *Pediatrics* **108** (2): 230–8. doi:10.1542/peds.108.2.230. PMID 11483782. http://pediatrics.aappublications.org/cgi/pmidlookup?view=long&pmid=11483782.

99. De Clercq E, Field HJ (2006). "Antiviral prodrugs - the development of successful prodrug strategies for antiviral chemotherapy". *Br. J. Pharmacol.* **147** (1): 1–11. doi:10.1038/sj.bjp.0706446. PMID 16284630.

100. Leung DT, Sacks SL. (2003). "Current treatment options to prevent perinatal transmission of herpes simplex virus". *Expert Opin. Pharmacother.* **4** (10): 1809–1819. doi:10.1517/14656566.4.10.1809. PMID 14521490.

101. The effects of antiviral therapy on the distribution of herpes simplex virus type 1 to ganglionic neurons and its consequences during, immediately following and several months after treatment"[1]"

102. Famciclovir and Valacyclovir Differ in the Prevention of Herpes Simplex Virus Type 1 Latency in Mice: a Quantitative Study"[2]"

103. Persistence of Infectious Herpes Simplex Virus Type 2 in the Nervous System in Mice after Antiviral Chemotherapy"[3]"

104. Observation May Indicate A Possible Clinical Effect On Latency"[4]"

105. Thackray AM, Field HJ. (1996). "Differential effects of famciclovir and valacyclovir on the pathogenesis of herpes simplex virus in a murine infection model including reactivation from latency". *J. Infect. Dis.* **173** (2): 291–299. PMID 8568288.

106. Worrall G (06 Jul 1996). "Evidence for efficacy of topical acyclovir in recurrent herpes labialis is weak". *BMJ* **313** (7048): 46. PMID 8664786. http://www.bmj.com/cgi/content/full/313/7048/46/a.

107. Spruance SL, Rea TL, Thoming C, Tucker R, Saltzman R, Boon R (1997). "Penciclovir cream for the treatment of herpes simplex labialis. A randomized, multicenter, double-blind, placebo-controlled trial. Topical Penciclovir Collaborative Study Group". *JAMA* **277** (17): 1374–9. doi:10.1001/jama.277.17.1374. PMID 9134943. http://jama.ama-assn.org/cgi/content/abstract/277/17/1374.

108. "Drug Name: ABREVA (docosanol) - approval". centerwatch.com. July 2000. http://www.centerwatch.com/patient/drugs/dru627.html. Retrieved on 2007-10-17.

109. "California Court Upholds Settlement Of Class Action Over Cold Sore Medicationl". BNA Inc.. July 2000. http://subscript.bna.com/SAMPLES/plp.nsf/85256269004a991e8525611300214487/29d5bb623a50fd25852572ad0074f772?OpenDocument. Retrieved on 2007-10-17.

110. Bishop, C.D. (1995). "Anti-viral Activity of the Essential Oil of Melaleuca alternifolia". Journal of Essential Oil Research: 641–644.

111. De Bony F, Tod M, Bidault R, On NT, Posner J, Rolan P. (2002). "Multiple interactions of cimetidine and probenecid with valacyclovir and its metabolite acyclovir". *Antimicrob. Agents Chemother.* **46** (2): 458–463. doi:10.1128/AAC.46.2.458-463.2002. PMID 11796358.

112. Karadi I, Karpati S, Romics L. (1998). "Aspirin in the management of recurrent herpes simplex virus infection". *Ann. Intern. Med.* **128** (8): 696–697. PMID 9537952.

113. Gebhardt BM, Varnell ED, Kaufman HE. (2004). "Acetylsalicylic acid reduces viral shedding induced by thermal stress". *Curr. Eye Res.* **29** (2-3): 119–125. doi:10.1080/02713680490504588. PMID 15512958.

114. "Herpevac Trial for Women". http://www.niaid.nih.gov/dmid/stds/herpevac/. Retrieved on 2008-02-25.

115. "Molecular Therapy - Abstract of article: 801. RNA Gene Therapy Targeting Herpes Simplex Virus". http://www.nature.com/mt/journal/v13/n1s/abs/mt2006942a.html.

116. Perfect MM, Bourne N, Ebel C, Rosenthal SL (2005). "Use of complementary and alternative medicine for the treatment of genital herpes". *Herpes* **12** (2): 38–41. PMID 16209859.

117. McCune MA, Perry HO, Muller SA, O'Fallon WM. (2005). "Treatment of recurrent herpes simplex infections with L-lysine monohydrochloride". *Cutis.* **34** (4): 366–373. PMID 6435961.

118. Griffith RS, Walsh DE, Myrmel KH, Thompson RW, Behforooz A. (1987). "Success of L-lysine therapy in frequently recurrent herpes simplex infection. Treatment and prophylaxis". *Dermatologica.* **175** (4): 183–190. PMID 3115841.

119. Griffith RS, Norins AL, Kagan C. (1978). "A multicentered study of lysine therapy in Herpes simplex infection". *Dermatologica.* **156** (5): 257–267. PMID 640102.

120. Vogler BK and Ernst E.. "Aloe vera: a systematic review of its clinical effectiveness.". *British Journal of General Practice* **49**: 823–828. http://www.jr2.ox.ac.uk/bandolier/booth/alternat/AT125.html.

121. Allahverdiyev A, Duran N, Ozguven M, Koltas S. (2004). "Antiviral activity of the volatile oils of Melissa officinalis L. against Herpes simplex virus type-2.". *Phytomedicine.* **11** (7-8): 657–661. doi:10.1016/j.phymed.2003.07.014. PMID 15636181.

122. Koytchev R, Alken RG, Dundarov S (1999). "Balm mint extract (Lo-701) for topical treatment of recurring herpes labialis". *Phytomedicine* **6** (4): 225–30. PMID 10589440.

123. Zacharopoulos VR, Phillips DM. (1997). "Vaginal formulations of carrageenan protect mice from herpes simplex virus infection". *Clin. Diagn. Lab. Immunol.* **4** (4): 465–468. PMID 9220165.

124. Carlucci MJ, Scolaro LA, Damonte EB. (1999). "Inhibitory action of natural carrageenans on Herpes simplex virus infection of mouse astrocytes". *Chemotherapy* **45** (6): 429–436. doi:10.1159/000007236. PMID 10567773.

125. Binns SE, Hudson J, Merali S, Arnason JT (2002). "Antiviral activity of characterized extracts from echinacea spp. (Heliantheae: Asteraceae) against herpes simplex virus (HSV-I)". *Planta Med.* **68** (9): 780–3. doi:10.1055/s-2002-34397. PMID 12357386.

126. Vonau B, Chard S, Mandalia S, Wilkinson D, Barton SE (2001). "Does the extract of the plant Echinacea purpurea influence the clinical course of recurrent genital herpes?". *Int J STD AIDS* **12** (3): 154–8. doi:10.1258/0956462 011916947. PMID 11231867.

127. Docherty JJ, Fu MM, Stiffler BS, Limperos RJ, Pokabla CM, DeLucia AL. (1999). "Resveratrol inhibition of herpes simplex virus replication". *Antiviral Res.* **43** (3): 145–155. doi:10.1016/S0166-3542(99)00042-X. PMID 10551373.

128. Docherty JJ, Smith JS, Fu MM, Stoner T, Booth T. (2004). "Effect of topically applied resveratrol on cutaneous herpes simplex virus infections in hairless mice". *Antiviral Res.* **61** (1): 19–26. doi:10.1016/j.antiviral.2003.07.001. PMID 14670590.

129. Weber ND, Andersen DO, North JA, Murray BK, Lawson LD, Hughes BG (1992). "In vitro virucidal effects of Allium sativum (garlic) extract and compounds". *Planta Med.* **58** (5): 417–23. doi:10.1055/s-2006-961504. PMID 1470664.

130. Chiu LC, Zhub W, Oo VE (2004). "A polysaccharide fraction from medicinal herb Prunella vulgaris downregulates the expression of herpes simplex virus antigen in Vero cells". *Journal of Ethnopharmacology* **93** (1): 63–68. doi:10.1016/j.jep.2004.03.024.

131. Andersen JH, Jenssen H, Gutteberg TJ. (2003). "Lactoferrin and lactoferricin inhibit Herpes simplex 1 and 2 infection and exhibit synergy when combined with acyclovir". *Antiviral Res.* **58** (3): 209–215. doi:10.1016/S0166-3542(02)00214-0. PMID 12767468.

132. Gaby AR (2006). "Natural remedies for Herpes simplex". *Altern Med Rev* **11** (2): 93–101. PMID 16813459.

133. Yazici AC, Baz K, Ikizoglu G (2006). "Recurrent herpes labialis during isotretinoin therapy: is there a role for photosensitivity?". *J Eur Acad Dermatol Venereol* **20** (1): 93–5. doi:10.1111/j.1468-3083.2005.01358.x. PMID 16405618.

134. Snipes W, Person S, Keith A, Cupp J (April 1975). "Butylated hydroxytoluene inactivated lipid-containing viruses". *Science* **188** (4183): 64–6. doi:10.1126/science.163494. PMID 163494. http://www.sciencemag.org/cgi/pmidlookup?view=long&pmid=163494.

135. Richards JT, Katz ME, Kern ER (October 1985). "Topical butylated hydroxytoluene treatment of genital herpes simplex virus infections of guinea pigs". *Antiviral Res.* **5** (5): 281–90. doi:10.1016/0166-3542(85)90042-7. PMID 2998276. http://linkinghub.elsevier.com/retrieve/pii/0166-3542(85)90042-7.

136. Vezina C, Steben M. (2001). "Genital Herpes: Psychosexual Impacts and Counselling" (PDF). The Canadian Journal of CME (June): 125–34. http://www.stacommunications.com/journals/cme/images/cmepdf/june01/hsv.pdf.

137. "HWerks.com Herpes Dating, HPV Dating, Information, Events and Support Community". http://www.HWerks.com.

138. "NationalHClub.com Local and National Herpes Events". http://www.NationalHClub.com.

139. "A to Z Herpes Support Groups". http://www.herpesaz.com/html/groups.html.

140. "Herpes Support Groups". http://www.herpes-coldsores.com/support/herpes.htm.

141. "Herpes Viruses Association". http://www.herpes.org.uk.

142. "Herpes & Cold Sore Support Forum". http://www.herpes-coldsores.com/messageforum.

143. "Herpes Dating H-Date.com - genital herpes dating/HPV picture". http://www.h-date.com.

144. "Herpes Dating, HPV Dating, and Support on Antopia's MPwH.net". http://www.mpwh.net/.

145. Green J, Ferrier S, Kocsis A, Shadrick J, Ukoumunne OC, Murphy S, Hetherton J. (2003). "Determinants of disclosure of genital herpes to partners.". *Sex. Transm. Infect.* **79** (1): 42–44. doi:10.1136/sti.79.1.42. PMID 12576613. http://sti.bmj.com/cgi/content/full/79/1/42.

GNU FREE DOCUMENTATION LICENSE

0. PREAMBLE

The purpose of this License is to make a manual, textbook, or other functional and useful document "free" in the sense of freedom: to assure everyone the effective freedom to copy and redistribute it, with or without modifying it, either commercially or noncommercially. Secondarily, this License preserves for the author and publisher a way to get credit for their work, while not being considered responsible for modifications made by others.

This License is a kind of "copyleft", which means that derivative works of the document must themselves be free in the same sense. It complements the GNU General Public License, which is a copyleft license designed for free software.

We have designed this License in order to use it for manuals for free software, because free software needs free documentation: a free program should come with manuals providing the same freedoms that the software does. But this License is not limited to software manuals; it can be used for any textual work, regardless of subject matter or whether it is published as a printed book. We recommend this License principally for works whose purpose is instruction or reference.

1. APPLICABILITY AND DEFINITIONS

This License applies to any manual or other work, in any medium, that contains a notice placed by the copyright holder saying it can be distributed under the terms of this License. Such a notice grants a world-wide, royalty-free license, unlimited in duration, to use that work under the conditions stated herein. The "Document", herein, refers to any such manual or work. Any member of the public is a licensee, and is addressed as "you". You accept the license if you copy, modify or distribute the work in a way requiring permission under copyright law.

A "Modified Version" of the Document means any work containing the Document or a portion of it, either copied verbatim, or with modifications and/or translated into another language.

A "Secondary Section" is a named appendix or a front-matter section of the Document that deals exclusively with the relationship of the publishers or authors of the Document to the Document's overall subject (or to related matters) and contains nothing that could fall directly within that overall subject. (Thus, if the Document is in part a textbook of mathematics, a Secondary Section may not explain any mathematics.) The relationship could be a matter of historical connection with the subject or with related matters, or of legal, commercial, philosophical, ethical or political position regarding them.

The "Invariant Sections" are certain Secondary Sections whose titles are designated, as being those of Invariant Sections, in the notice that says that the Document is released under this License. If a section does not fit the above definition of Secondary then it is not allowed to be designated as Invariant. The Document may contain zero Invariant Sections. If the Document does not identify any Invariant Sections then there are none.

The "Cover Texts" are certain short passages of text that are listed, as Front-Cover Texts or Back-Cover Texts, in the notice that says that the Document is released under this License. A Front-Cover Text may be at most 5 words, and a Back-Cover Text may be at most 25 words.

A "Transparent" copy of the Document means a machine-readable copy, represented in a format whose specification is available to the general public, that is suitable for revising the document straightforwardly with generic text editors or (for images composed of pixels) generic paint programs or (for drawings) some widely available drawing editor, and that is suitable for input to text formatters or for automatic translation to a variety of formats suitable for input to text formatters. A copy made in an otherwise Transparent file format whose markup, or absence of markup, has been arranged to thwart or discourage subsequent modification by readers is not Transparent. An image format is not Transparent if used for any substantial amount of text. A copy that is not "Transparent" is called "Opaque".

Examples of suitable formats for Transparent copies include plain ASCII without markup, Texinfo input format, LaTeX input format, SGML or XML using a publicly available DTD, and standard-conforming simple HTML, PostScript or PDF designed for human modification. Examples of transparent image formats include PNG, XCF and JPG. Opaque formats include proprietary formats that can be read and edited only by proprietary word processors, SGML or XML for which the DTD and/or processing tools are not generally available, and the machine-generated HTML, PostScript or PDF produced by some word processors for output purposes only.

The "Title Page" means, for a printed book, the title page itself, plus such following pages as are needed to hold, legibly, the material this License requires to appear in the title page. For works in formats which do not have any title page as such, "Title Page" means the text near the most prominent appearance of the work's title, preceding the beginning of the body of the text.

A section "Entitled XYZ" means a named subunit of the Document whose title either is precisely XYZ or contains XYZ in parentheses following text that translates XYZ in another language. (Here XYZ stands for a specific section name mentioned below, such as "Acknowledgements", "Dedications", "Endorsements", or "History".) To "Preserve the Title" of such a section when you modify the Document means that it remains a section "Entitled XYZ" according to this definition.

The Document may include Warranty Disclaimers next to the notice which states that this License applies to the Document. These Warranty Disclaimers are considered to be included by reference in this License, but only as regards disclaiming warranties: any other implication that these Warranty Disclaimers may have is void and has no effect on the meaning of this License.

2. VERBATIM COPYING

You may copy and distribute the Document in any medium, either commercially or noncommercially, provided that this License, the copyright notices, and the license notice saying this License applies to the Document are reproduced in all copies, and that you add no other conditions whatsoever to those of this License. You may not use technical measures to obstruct or control the reading or further copying of the copies you make or distribute. However, you may accept compensation in exchange for copies. If you distribute a large enough number of copies you must also follow the conditions in section 3.

You may also lend copies, under the same conditions stated above, and you may publicly display copies.

3. COPYING IN QUANTITY

If you publish printed copies (or copies in media that commonly have printed covers) of the Document, numbering more than 100, and the Document's license notice requires Cover Texts, you must enclose the copies in covers that carry, clearly and legibly, all these Cover Texts: Front-Cover Texts on the front cover, and Back-Cover Texts on the back cover. Both covers must also clearly and legibly identify you as the publisher of these copies. The front cover must present the full title with all words of the title equally prominent and visible. You may add other material on the covers in addition. Copying with changes limited to the covers, as long as they preserve the title of the Document and satisfy these conditions, can be treated as verbatim copying in other respects.

If the required texts for either cover are too voluminous to fit legibly, you should put the first ones listed (as many as fit reasonably) on the actual cover, and continue the rest onto adjacent pages.

If you publish or distribute Opaque copies of the Document numbering more than 100, you must either include a machine-readable Transparent copy along with each Opaque copy, or state in or with each Opaque copy a computer-network location from which the general network-using public has access to download using public-standard network protocols a complete Transparent copy of the Document, free of added material. If you use the latter option, you must take reasonably prudent steps, when you begin distribution of Opaque copies in quantity, to ensure that this Transparent copy will remain thus accessible at the stated location until at least one year after the last time you distribute an Opaque copy (directly or through your agents or retailers) of that edition to the public.

It is requested, but not required, that you contact the authors of the Document well before redistributing any large number of copies, to give them a chance to provide you with an updated version of the Document.

4. MODIFICATIONS

You may copy and distribute a Modified Version of the Document under the conditions of sections 2 and 3 above, provided that you release the Modified Version under precisely this License, with the Modified Version filling the role of the Document, thus licensing distribution and modification of the Modified Version to whoever possesses a copy of it. In addition, you must do these things in the Modified Version:

A. Use in the Title Page (and on the covers, if any) a title distinct from that of the Document, and from those of previous versions (which should, if there were any, be listed in the History section of the Document). You may use the same title as a previous version if the original publisher of that version gives permission.

B. List on the Title Page, as authors, one or more persons or entities responsible for authorship of the modifications in the Modified Version, together with at least five of the principal authors of the Document (all of its principal authors, if it has fewer than five), unless they release you from this requirement.

C. State on the Title page the name of the publisher of the Modified Version, as the publisher.

D. Preserve all the copyright notices of the Document.

E. Add an appropriate copyright notice for your modifications adjacent to the other copyright notices.

F. Include, immediately after the copyright notices, a license notice giving the public permission to use the Modified Version under the terms of this License, in the form shown in the Addendum below.

G. Preserve in that license notice the full lists of Invariant Sections and required Cover Texts given in the Document's license notice.

H. Include an unaltered copy of this License.

I. Preserve the section Entitled "History", Preserve its Title, and add to it an item stating at least the title, year, new authors, and publisher of the Modified Version as given on the Title Page. If there is no section Entitled "History" in the Document, create one stating the title, year, authors, and publisher of the Document as given on its Title Page, then add an item describing the Modified Version as stated in the previous sentence.

J. Preserve the network location, if any, given in the Document for public access to a Transparent copy of the Document, and likewise the network locations given in the Document for previous versions it was based on. These may be placed in the "History" section. You may omit a network location for a work that was published at least four years before the Document itself, or if the original publisher of the version it refers to gives permission.

K. For any section entitled "Acknowledgements" or "Dedications", Preserve the Title of the section, and preserve in the section all the substance and tone of each of the contributor acknowledgements and/or dedications given therein.

L. Preserve all the Invariant Sections of the Document, unaltered in their text and in their titles. Section numbers or the equivalent are not considered part of the section titles.

M. Delete any section entitled "Endorsements". Such a section may not be included in the Modified Version.

N. Do not retitle any existing section to be entitled "Endorsements" or to conflict in title with any Invariant Section.

O. Preserve any Warranty Disclaimers.

If the Modified Version includes new front-matter sections or appendices that qualify as Secondary Sections and contain no material copied from the Document, you may at your option designate some or all of these sections as Invariant. To do this, add their titles to the list of Invariant Sections in the Modified Version's license notice. These titles must be distinct from any other section titles.

You may add a section entitled "Endorsements", provided it contains nothing but endorsements of your Modified Version by various parties—for example, statements of peer review or that the text has been approved by an organization as the authoritative definition of a standard.

You may add a passage of up to five words as a Front-Cover Text, and a passage of up to 25 words as a Back-Cover Text, to the end of the list of Cover Texts in the Modified Version. Only one passage of Front-Cover Text and one of Back-Cover Text may be added by (or through arrangements made by) any one entity. If the Document already includes a Cover Text for the same cover, previously added by you or by arrangement made by the same entity you are acting on behalf of, you may not add another; but you may replace the old one, on explicit permission from the previous publisher that added the old one.

The author(s) and publisher(s) of the Document do not by this License give permission to use their names for publicity for or to assert or imply endorsement of any Modified Version.

5. COMBINING DOCUMENTS

You may combine the Document with other documents released under this License, under the terms defined in section 4 above for modified versions, provided that you include in the combination all of the Invariant Sections of all of the original documents, unmodified, and list them all as Invariant Sections of your combined work in its license notice, and that you preserve all their Warranty Disclaimers.

The combined work need only contain one copy of this License, and multiple identical Invariant Sections may be replaced with a single copy. If there are multiple Invariant Sections with the same name but different contents, make the title of each such section unique by adding at the end of it, in parentheses, the name of the original author or publisher of that section if known, or else a unique number. Make the same adjustment to the section titles in the list of Invariant Sections in the license notice of the combined work.

In the combination, you must combine any sections entitled "History" in the various original documents, forming one section entitled "History";

likewise combine any sections entitled "Acknowledgements", and any sections entitled "Dedications". You must delete all sections entitled "Endorsements."

6. COLLECTIONS OF DOCUMENTS

You may make a collection consisting of the Document and other documents released under this License, and replace the individual copies of this License in the various documents with a single copy that is included in the collection, provided that you follow the rules of this License for verbatim copying of each of the documents in all other respects.

You may extract a single document from such a collection, and distribute it individually under this License, provided you insert a copy of this License into the extracted document, and follow this License in all other respects regarding verbatim copying of that document.

7. AGGREGATION WITH INDEPENDENT WORKS

A compilation of the Document or its derivatives with other separate and independent documents or works, in or on a volume of a storage or distribution medium, is called an "aggregate" if the copyright resulting from the compilation is not used to limit the legal rights of the compilation's users beyond what the individual works permit. When the Document is included in an aggregate, this License does not apply to the other works in the aggregate which are not themselves derivative works of the Document.

If the Cover Text requirement of section 3 is applicable to these copies of the Document, then if the Document is less than one half of the entire aggregate, the Document's Cover Texts may be placed on covers that bracket the Document within the aggregate, or the electronic equivalent of covers if the Document is in electronic form. Otherwise they must appear on printed covers that bracket the whole aggregate.

8. TRANSLATION

Translation is considered a kind of modification, so you may distribute translations of the Document under the terms of section 4. Replacing Invariant Sections with translations requires special permission from their copyright holders, but you may include translations of some or all Invariant Sections in addition to the original versions of these Invariant Sections. You may include a translation of this License, and all the license notices in the Document, and any Warranty Disclaimers, provided that you also include the original English version of this License and the original versions of those notices and disclaimers. In case of a disagreement between the translation and the original version of this License or a notice or disclaimer, the original version will prevail.

If a section in the Document is entitled "Acknowledgements", "Dedications", or "History", the requirement (section 4) to Preserve its Title (section 1) will typically require changing the actual title.

9. TERMINATION

You may not copy, modify, sublicense, or distribute the Document except as expressly provided for under this License. Any other attempt to copy, modify, sublicense or distribute the Document is void, and will automatically terminate your rights under this License. However, parties who have received copies, or rights, from you under this License will not have their licenses terminated so long as such parties remain in full compliance.

10. FUTURE REVISIONS OF THIS LICENSE

The Free Software Foundation may publish new, revised versions of the GNU Free Documentation License from time to time. Such new versions will be similar in spirit to the present version, but may differ in detail to address new problems or concerns. See http://www.gnu.org/copyleft/.

Each version of the License is given a distinguishing version number. If the Document specifies that a particular numbered version of this License "or any later version" applies to it, you have the option of following the terms and conditions either of that specified version or of any later version that has been published (not as a draft) by the Free Software Foundation. If the Document does not specify a version number of this License, you may choose any version ever published (not as a draft) by the Free Software Foundation.

INDEX

www.ingramcontent.com/pod-product-compliance
Lightning Source LLC
Chambersburg PA
CBHW071229290326
41931CB00037B/2534